T0228319

Civic Engagement
and the Baby Boomer
Generation
Research, Policy, and Practice
Perspectives

THE HAWORTH PRESS
Titles of Related Interest

Volunteerism in Geriatric Settings edited by Vera R. Jackson

Volunteerism Marketing: New Vistas for Nonprofit and Public Sector Management edited by Donald R. Self and Walter W. Wymer Jr.

University-Community Partnerships: Universities in Civic Engagement edited by Tracy M. Soska and Alice K. Johnson Butterfield

Educating Students to Make a Difference: Community-Based Service Learning edited by Joseph R. Ferrari and Judith G. Chapman

Spiritual Wisdom for Successful Retirement: Living Forward by C. W. Brister

Adventures in Senior Living: Learning How to Make Retirement Meaningful and Enjoyable by Rev. J. Lawrence Driskill

Advancing Aging Policy as the 21st Century Begins edited by Francis G. Caro, Robert Morris, and Jill R. Norton

Challenges of Aging on U.S. Families: Policy and Practice Implications edited by Richard K. Caputo

Civic Engagement and the Baby Boomer Generation

Research, Policy, and Practice Perspectives

Laura B. Wilson, PhD
Sharon P. Simson, PhD
Editors

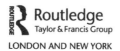

Routledge
Taylor & Francis Group

LONDON AND NEW YORK

Transferred to Digital Printing 2008 by Routledge 2008
2 Park Square, Milton Park, Abingdon, Oxon, OX14 4RN
270 Madison Ave, New York NY 10016

For more information on this book or to order, visit
http://www.haworthpress.com/store/product.asp?sku=5700

or call 1-800-HAWORTH (800-429-6784) in the United States and Canada
or (607) 722-5857 outside the United States and Canada

or contact orders@HaworthPress.com

© 2006 by The Haworth Press, Inc. All rights reserved. No part of this work may be reproduced or
utilized in any form or by any means, electronic or mechanical, including photocopying, microfilm,
and recording, or by any information storage and retrieval system, without permission in writing
from the publisher.

The Haworth Press, Inc., 10 Alice Street, Binghamton, NY 13904-1580.

PUBLISHER'S NOTE
The development, preparation, and publication of this work has been undertaken with great care.
However, the Publisher, employees, editors, and agents of The Haworth Press are not responsible
for any errors contained herein or for consequences that may ensue from use of materials or information contained in this work. The Haworth Press is committed to the dissemination of ideas and information according to the highest standards of intellectual freedom and the free exchange of ideas.
Statements made and opinions expressed in this publication do not necessarily reflect the views of
the Publisher, Directors, management, or staff of The Haworth Press, Inc., or an endorsement by
them.

Cover design by Kerry E. Mack.

Library of Congress Cataloging-in-Publication Data

Civic engagement and the baby boomer generation : research, policy, and practice perspectives /
Laura B. Wilson, Sharon P. Simson, editors.
    p. cm.
Includes bibliographical references and index.
ISBN-13: 978-0-7890-0551-9 (hc. : alk. paper)
ISBN-10: 0-7890-0551-4 (hc. : alk. paper)
ISBN-13: 978-0-7890-0578-6 (pbk. : alk. paper)
ISBN-10: 0-7890-0578-6 (pbk. : alk. paper)

1. Social participation—United States. 2. Baby boom generation—United States. 3. Baby boom
generation—Retirement—United States. 4. Older volunteers—United States. 5. Older people—
Education (Continuing education)—United States. I. Wilson, Laura B. II. Simson, Sharon.

HN59.2.C54 2005
305.244'0973—dc22

                                                                    2005017541

CONTENTS

ABOUT THE EDITORS

Laura B. Wilson, PhD, is Director of the Center on Aging and Professor of Public and Community Health at the University of Maryland, College Park. She has been Principal Investigator on a variety of national and international research, demonstration, and training projects related to civic engagement and the fifty-plus population, including the National Eldercare Institute on Employment and Volunteerism, AmeriCorps T/TA National Provider for Home-Based Care and Independent Living, the Legacy Leadership Institutes, AmeriCorps National Direct: Legacy Corps for Health and Independent Living, and Legacy Corps for Multi-Generational Service. Legacy Corps has been presented with the 2005 Archstone Award by the American Public Health Association Gerontological Health Section for innovation in translating research into practice. Dr. Wilson is Director of RSVPI: Retired and Senior Volunteer Program International and a fellow of the Gerontological Society of America.

Sharon P. Simson, PhD, is Research Professor at the University of Maryland Center on Aging and Coordinator of Legacy College for Lifelong Learning, the Graduate Gerontology Certificate Program, and the Legacy Leadership Institute on Humor Practices. She is Editor with Laura B. Wilson of the Community Gerontology Series (Haworth), *Aging and Prevention* (Haworth), the *Handbook of Geriatric Emergency Care,* and *Minority Health and Aging.* She is Senior Editor of *Horticulture as Therapy: Principles and Practice* (Haworth). Dr. Simson is Chairperson of the Maryland State Unit of Action for Healthy Kids. She is a fellow in Retirement Housing of the American Association of Homes and Services for the Aged.

CONTRIBUTORS

Kwofie Danso, MSW, is a doctoral student at the College of Social Work, Ohio State University. He was a research associate at the Center for Social Development, Washington University. His research interests include civic engagement, international development, decentralization, and NGO-government partnerships for development.

William A. Galston, PhD, is Professor, School of Public Affairs, University of Maryland at College Park, and director of the university's Institute for Philosophy and Public Policy. He is also the founding director of CIRCLE (the Center for Information and Research on Civic Learning and Engagement), funded by the Pew Charitable Trusts. From January 1993 through May 1995 Dr. Galston served as deputy assistant to President Clinton for Domestic Policy. He is the author of six books and nearly 100 articles dealing with political and moral philosophy, American politics, and public policy.

Richard Goff is a PhD candidate in history at the University of Pittsburgh. He received his master's degree in history from Eastern Michigan University. He is adjunct faculty at Chatham College where he teaches American social history. He has served as graduate advisory editor for *Social Science History* and is currently the editorial assistant for the *Journal of Intergenerational Relationships.*

Karen Harlow-Rosentraub, PhD, is associate professor, Frances Payne Bolton School of Nursing, Case Western Reserve University. Dr. Harlow has directed the evaluation component of Legacy Corps for Health and Independent Living for the University of Maryland Center on Aging for the past two years. She has published in numerous journals such as *Nonprofit Sector Research Quarterly, Journal of Urban Affairs, The Gerontologist, Journal of Applied Gerontology,* and *Urban Affairs Quarterly.*

Jim Hinterlong, PhD, is Assistant Professor at the School of Social Work and an affiliate of the Pepper Institute on Aging and Public Policy at Florida State University. He is also a faculty associate of the

Global Service Institute at Washington University in St. Louis and a Hartford Geriatric Social Work Faculty Scholar. His scholarly interests include the impact of demographic change on public policy formulation, especially with respect to the promotion of productive engagement in later life through volunteerism, service, caregiving, and paid employment.

Mark H. Lopez, PhD, is the research director at CIRCLE (the Center for Information and Research on Civic Learning and Engagement) and a research assistant professor at the University of Maryland School of Public Affairs. He holds a PhD in economics from Princeton University.

Tracey T. Manning, PhD, is Research Associate Professor at the University of Maryland's Center on Aging. She conducts leadership research and development for the center's Legacy Leadership Institutes. She has a joint appointment with the university's Academy of Leadership where she directs a longitudinal study of adolescent leadership and social responsibility. Formerly professor of psychology at the College of Notre Dame of Maryland, Dr. Manning writes and consults on transformational leadership development and assessment.

Amanda Moore McBride, PhD, is Assistant Professor at the George Warren Brown School of Social Work and research director in the Center for Social Development, Washington University in St. Louis. She is coprincipal investigator with Michael Sherraden for the Global Service Institute's research agenda. Her scholarship focuses on the forms of civic engagement and civic service worldwide, civic effects of asset building, and developmental effects of civic service.

Sally Newman, PhD, is Emerita Professor at the University of Pittsburgh and founder and former executive director of Generations Together. She is founding chair of the International Consortium for Intergenerational Programs (ICIP) and founding editor of the *Journal of Intergenerational Relationships* (JIR), a quarterly journal of The Haworth Press, Inc. Dr. Newman has edited two books on intergenerational studies and has been a lecturer and researcher in the intergenerational field in the United States and abroad since the 1970s.

Robert D. Putnam is Peter and Isabel Malkin Professor of Public Policy. He teaches graduate courses at the Kennedy School and undergraduate courses at the Faculty of Arts and Sciences. He is a member of the National Academy of Sciences, a Fellow of the British Academy, and past president of the American Political Science Association. Raised in a small town in the Midwest and educated at Swarthmore, Oxford, and Yale, he has served as Dean of the Kennedy School of Government. He has written a dozen books, translated into seventeen languages, including the best-selling *Bowling Alone: The Collapse and Revival of American Community* and, more recently, *Better Together: Restoring the American Community,* a study of promising new forms of social connectedness. He founded the Saguaro Seminar, bringing together leading thinkers and practitioners to develop actionable ideas for civic renewal. He is now studying the challenges of building community in an increasingly diverse society.

David B. Rymph, PhD, trained as a cultural anthropologist, has spent his thirty-year public service career primarily in the areas of program evaluation, research, and policy development. He has worked at the local, state, national, and international levels. Dr. Rymph retired in 2003 from federal service where he worked for the Peace Corps, U.S. HUD, ACTION, and the Corporation for National and Community Service. He now lives in Port Townsend, Washington, and continues to do consulting and training on national service issues.

Thomas H. Sander, JD, is Executive Director of the Saguaro Seminar. Prior to taking this position, he was director of the Fund for Social Entrepreneurs at Youth Service America and served as a senior policy advisor on national service for the U.S. Senate's Labor and Human Resources Committee where he played a major role in the enactment of the 1993 National Service Trust Act. He has worked as a management consultant at Bain and Company and assisted Harvard University's president in negotiating and consummating some of the first debt for education swaps in the world. He received a JD from the Harvard Law School.

Priyanthi Silva, PhD, was a senior analyst on the Senior Corps Futures Study for the Corporation for National and Community Service that provided the data for Chapter 3 in this book. She obtained her PhD in gerontology from the University of Massachusetts, Boston. She is currently a research analyst at Westat, a survey research organization based in Rockville, Maryland. She has worked on gender identity styles of women, elder abuse, volunteering, and other aging-related studies.

Ben H. Slijkhuis became director of the Netherlands Platform Older People and Europe in 2002 after extensive experience in social, educational, and international activities. He served as director of EXIS, the Dutch national organization for international youth activities and policies, vice president of Eriyca, the European Youth Information and Counselling Association, and head of the International Centre of NIZW, the Netherlands Institute for Care and Welfare, and a policy advisor for the Ministry of Social Affairs and Employment.

Jack Steele, MA, is the project director of Legacy Corps and co-director of Retired and Senior Volunteer Programs International for the Center on Aging at the University of Maryland. He has spent over twenty years developing and administering aging services programs and working in the volunteer sector. He has worked with nonprofit, governmental, and faith-based organizations to develop innovative volunteer programs for older adults both nationally and internationally.

Fengyan Tang, MA, MSW, is a PhD candidate at the George Warren Brown School of Social Work, Washington University in St. Louis. Her areas of interest are gerontology, particularly in social policy, volunteering, productive aging, and civic engagement.

Cynthia Thomas, PhD, directed the Senior Corps Futures Study for the Corporation for National and Community Service, on which Chapter 3 is based. Dr. Thomas is a senior study director at Westat and an associate professor at Albert Einstein College of Medicine. She has studied the use of health care services and health and aging, elder abuse, and other topics related to older adults. At Westat she directs large-scale survey research studies in these and other fields.

Joke M. Zwart is policy officer for the Netherlands Platform Older People and Europe and secretary of AGE Platform Netherlands, a platform of forty Dutch NGOs working for and with older people that exchange information about EU policy developments relevant to the older people's sector.

Preface

Civic engagement presents a powerful opportunity and exciting challenge to both the generation of baby boomers who are coming of age in the next several decades and to nonprofit organizations seeking to meet their volunteer needs. Unlike any previous generation, the baby boomers, born between 1946-1964, are defying stereotypes about aging while seeking new and meaningful lifestyles. They enjoy increased longevity, better health, higher educational attainment, and more discretionary income. The first wave of boomers, 77 million strong, began to turn fifty-five in the year 2001. By the year 2020, there will be 69 million persons age sixty-five and over and they will account for over 20 percent of the total U.S. population (Treas, 1995). They are active individuals who have amassed considerable expertise, experience, and skills while making valuable contributions to all sectors of society: business and industry, government, the military, education, religion, family, and community.

This new generation of older adults expects much from the next chapters of their lives. Shaped by a variety of shared historical experiences, the boomers reflect distinct life values that directly impact their expectations about their futures. They eschew retirement and view their later years as opportunities to continue and increase their contributions to society by exploring new options, continuing life-long learning, working in new capacities, participating in sophisticated volunteer activities, and engaging in meaningful civic pursuits (Independent Sector, 1989; Keefe, 2001; Moody, 2000; Nordstrom, 2004; Wilson & Simson, 2002; Wilson, Steele, D'heron, & Thompson, 2002).

Despite the documented overall decline in civic engagement in our society, the baby boomer generation holds the promise of continuing to generate social capital through engagement in civic affairs (Putnam, 2000; Wilson et al., 2002). The purpose of this book is to enhance civic engagement by presenting current, state-of-the-art research, policy, and practice perspectives about civic engagement and the baby boomer generation. This book seeks to provide an integrated perspective regarding current knowledge and thinking on this topic by

1. establishing, integrating, and communicating a foundation of knowledge about civic engagement of the baby boomer generation;
2. presenting the latest research and evaluation studies of civic engagement of the baby boomer generation that can be used by others to develop programs, policy, and research related to civic engagement for all ages;
3. presenting best practice models of civic engagement by the baby boomer generation that can be replicated by other age cohorts and programs;
4. demonstrating the contributions and implications of civic engagement by the baby boomer generation to public policy on local, national, and global levels;
5. encouraging institutions, professionals, communities, and citizens to recognize the impact of the baby boomer generation on civic engagement in order to utilize most effectively their skills and commitment to enhancing social capital;
6. defining an agenda for future policy, research, and practice related to civic engagement by the baby boomer generation;
7. increasing civic engagement by the baby boomer generation in their communities, government, health services, older adult programs and initiatives, civic associations, faith-based organizations, youth programs and schools, and other civic undertakings;
8. mending the decline of civic engagement among younger people by showing the civic engagement legacies of the baby boomer generation in terms of developing social capital through their attitudes, values, commitment, and activities; and
9. promoting understanding of civic engagement programs, policy agendas, and opportunities on local, national, and global levels.

Civic Engagement and the Baby Boomer Generation: Research, Policy, and Practice Perspectives contains twelve chapters organized into five sections:

Part I: Overview of Civic Engagement
Part II: National Service and the Fifty-Plus Population

Part III: Lifelong Learning and Civic Engagement
Part IV: Intergenerational Concepts and Applications
Part V: National and Global Agendas

Contributors are recognized experts who have advanced civic engagement through their research, policy work, and best practice models. They are pioneers in focusing attention on the importance, value, and centrality of civic engagement to creating the vital social capital of a civil society. It is our hope that this book will provide readers with new perspectives that will empower them to enhance civic engagement, locally, nationally, and globally, today and tomorrow.

REFERENCES

Independent Sector. (1989). *Giving and Volunteering in the United States.* Washington, DC: Independent Sector.

Keefe, S. (2001). *Tapping Senior Power-Community Partnerships That Work.* Washington, DC: Corporation for National Service.

Moody, H. R. (2000). *Aging: Concepts and Controversies.* Thousand Oaks, CA: Pine Forge Press.

Nordstrom, N. M. (2004). *EIN Monthly Newsletter.* Elderhostel Institute. Available online at http://www.elderhostel.org.

Putnam, R. (2000). *Bowling Alone.* New York: Simon and Schuster.

Treas, J. (1995). Older Americans in the 1990s and Beyond. *Population Bulletin,* 50(2).

Wilson, L. B. & Simson, S. (2002). *Next Chapters Retirement Planning for the Baby Boomers.* College Park, MD: University of Maryland Center on Aging.

Wilson, L. B., Steele, J., D'heron, C., & Thompson, E. (2002). The Leadership Institute for Active Aging: A Volunteer Recruitment and Retention Model. *Journal of Volunteer Administration,* (20)2: 28-36.

Acknowledgments

With appreciation to our colleagues at the Haworth Press: Bill Cohen (Publisher), Bill Palmer (Vice President & Publications Director), Patricia Brown (Editorial Production Manager), Chris Corey (Royalties Manager), Jennifer Durgan (Production Editor), Dawn Krisko (Senior Production Editor), Kerry E. Mack (Cover Designer), Mary Beth Madden (Copy Editor), Peg Marr (Senior Production Editor), Sandi Raub (Typesetter), Joshua Ribakove (Manager, Advertising Copywriting), Tracy F. Sayles (Assistant Production Editor, Book Division), Sandra Jones Sickels (Vice President, Marketing), Margaret Tatich (Sales and Publicity Manager), Jason Wint (Art Production Assistant).

With gratitude to the faculty and staff of the University of Maryland Center on Aging and especially to Louise Benas, Coordinator.

In memoriam: Stuart K. Wilson, MD, and Nancy E. Pastor.

PART I:
OVERVIEW OF CIVIC ENGAGEMENT

Chapter 1

Civic Engagement in the United States

William A. Galston
Mark H. Lopez

INTRODUCTION

Although the United States is a stable constitutional democracy, worries about the condition of U.S. civic life are widespread. Scholars, elected officials, and ordinary citizens are concerned about the apparent weakening of civil society as well as documented declines in political activities such as voting. The purpose of this chapter is not to advocate specific public policies, but rather to summarize what is known about the condition of civic life in the United States. Survey data will provide the principal evidence for our conclusions.

We begin, however, by offering a more precise definition of the phenomenon we seek to measure. We may divide the broad concept of "civic life" into two main parts: participation in official politics, through activities such as voting, working for candidates and campaigns, and writing letters to the editor about political issues; and second, engagement in a range of voluntary sector activities and organizations such as sports leagues, garden clubs, and local civic associations.

The relation between these two dimensions of civic life is complex and contestable. In some circumstances, and for some population groups, they are mutually supportive; more of one seems to yield more of the other. For other groups in different circumstances, participation in one aspect of civic life may come at the expense of participation in the other. (Something of this sort appears to be happening among significant numbers of young adults today.)

WHY DOES CIVIC DISENGAGEMENT MATTER?

Before we proceed to measure our civic life, we must ask why it matters, and why we should care if statistics suggest that it is weakening. Let us begin with a truism about representative democracy: political engagement is not sufficient for political effectiveness, but it is necessary. If today's disengaged citizens have legitimate interests that do not wholly coincide with the interests of participators, those interests cannot shape public decisions unless they are forcefully articulated. The withdrawal of a cohort of citizens from public affairs disturbs the balance of public deliberation, to the detriment of those who withdraw (and many others besides).

Second, there is an old-fashioned argument for obligation. All Americans derive great benefits from their membership in a stable, prosperous, and free society. These goods do not fall like manna from heaven; they must be produced, and renewed, by each generation. Every citizen has a moral responsibility to contribute his or her fair share to sustaining the public institutions and processes on which we all depend, and from which we all benefit.

We come, third, to the relation between citizenship and self-development. Even if we agree (and we may not) on the activities that constitute good citizenship, one may still wonder why it is good to be a good citizen. After all, it is possible for many individuals to realize their good in ways that do not involve the active exercise of citizenship. Even if we accept Aristotle's characterization of politics as the architectonic activity, it does not follow that the development of civic capacities is architectonic for every soul.

Still, there is something to the proposition that under appropriate circumstances, political engagement helps develop capacities that are intrinsically important. We have in mind the sorts of intellectual and moral capacities that Tocqueville and John Stuart Mill discuss, or gesture toward: among them—enlarged interests, a wider human sympathy, a sense of active responsibility for oneself, the skills needed to work with others toward goods that can only be obtained or created through collective action, and the powers of sympathetic understanding needed to build bridges of persuasive words to those with whom one must act.

These links between participation and character development are empirical, not theoretical, propositions, and we do not (yet) have the kind of evidence we need to sustain them against doubt. On the other hand, we do not have compelling reasons to doubt them, and they can at least be advanced as a not-implausible profession of public faith— as long as we are not too categorical about it.

It may well be that even as civic engagement has declined, it has become not less but more necessary for the development of the human capacities just sketched. Underlying this conjecture is the suspicion that as the market has become more pervasive during the past generation as organizing metaphor and as daily experience, the range of opportunities to develop nonmarket skills and dispositions has narrowed. For various reasons, the solidaristic organizations that dominated the U.S. landscape from the 1930s through the early 1960s have weakened, and the principle of individual choice has emerged as our central value. Indeed, citizenship itself has become optional, as the sense of civic obligation (to vote, or for that matter to do anything else of civic consequence) has faded and as the military draft has been replaced by all-volunteer armed forces. When the chips are down we prefer exit to voice, and any sense of loyalty to something larger than ourselves has all but disappeared. In this context, the experience of collective action directed toward common purposes is one of the few conceivable counterweights to today's hyperextended principle of individual choice.

A focus of this chapter is a series of comparisons among different age cohorts in the U.S. population. It is important, however, not to leap to the conclusion that differences among age cohorts is solely, or even mainly, the result of different positions in the life cycle. On the contrary: political scientists and sociologists have identified the specific formative experiences of young adults as sources of outlooks and behaviors that they carry with them for the remainder of their lives. For example, the generation of Americans that came of age between the late 1920s and mid-1940s was decisively shaped by the Great Depression and World War II. These Americans tend to be more participatory and less individualistic in their outlook than are their younger fellow citizens. As the presidential election of 2004 demonstrated, Americans who came of age during the controversy over Vietnam are marked for life by the sides they took during that tumultuous era. There is preliminary evidence that young Americans who came to maturity during the economic expansion and post–Cold War tranquility of the 1990s express more confidence in government and are more optimistic than their older brothers and sisters.

With these introductory comments as background, we turn now to an empirical analysis of U.S. civic life. We divide this assessment into two parts: civic attitudes and knowledge and civic behavior.

CIVIC ATTITUDES AND KNOWLEDGE

The citizens of the United States remain deeply committed to what many call the "American creed," an amalgam of constitutional democracy in politics, equal opportunity in the economy, and freedom in society. According to a much-cited survey conducted by the University of Virginia's Post-Modernity Project, support for the basic elements of the creed runs in excess of 90 percent in the population as a whole and in key subgroups (Post-Modernity Project, 1996). Decades before the events of September 11, 2001, and continuing up to the present, overwhelming majorities have consistently expressed pride in their country.[1]

Evidence suggests, however, that young adults are somewhat less committed to the American creed than are their parents and grandparents. Through the 1990s, surveys suggested that young people were significantly less likely than their adult counterparts to say that the United States is the greatest country, that its system of government is the best possible, that they are proud to live under that system, or that they would rather live in the United States than in other countries.[2] Futhermore, today's high school seniors are less likely to agree that despite its many faults, our system of doing things is still the best in the world than was the previous generation. In 1977, two-thirds of high school seniors agreed with this statement; by 2000, agreement had fallen significantly, to only 55 percent (Zill, 2002). Although numerous surveys have shown a surge in patriotism among young people in the wake of September 11, 2001, the most recent evidence suggests that this phenomenon may be short-lived.

Moral Evaluations of the United States

Evidence suggests that increasing numbers of Americans perceive their society to be suffering a moral decline. A half century ago, more than 50 percent of Americans responded affirmatively when asked,

"Do you think people in general lead as good lives—honest and moral—as they used to?" As recent as the mid-1960s, more than 40 percent agreed. By 1998, that figure had declined to 28 percent (Putnam, 2000). By 2002, it had fallen even further, to only 21 percent (Pew Research Center, 2002, question 2).

This perception of moral decline is especially pronounced in citizens' evaluations of young people. When asked "Do you think that young people today have as strong a sense of right and wrong as they did, say, fifty years ago?" 57 percent answered affirmatively in 1952, and 41 percent as recently as 1965. Today, that figure has bottomed out at only 19 percent (Pew Research Center, 2002, question 3).

Attitudes Toward Government

Over the past two generations, Americans' trust in the national government has declined sharply. In the early 1960s, about three-quarters of U.S. citizens trusted the national government to do what is right all or most of the time. By the mid-1990s, only one-quarter did. In the second half of the 1990s, trust in government increased modestly, to nearly 40 percent, before the Clinton scandals knocked it down again.[3] September 11, 2001, produced a surge in trust in government, which has since subsided, although trust remains significantly higher than before the terrorist attacks. Trust in the legislative and executive branches declined about equally, while trust in the judiciary remained stable. Trust in state and local government also declined but is consistently higher than is trust in the national government.

Through the past decade, scholars in the United States have debated the cause of this historic shift. The most comprehensive exploration reached the following conclusions.

1. The early 1960s probably represented a period of abnormally high trust, because the World War II generation, with its positive experiences of government, was demographically and politically dominant.

2. Key events of the mid-1960s through the early 1970s—Vietnam, Watergate, domestic disruption, and the surge in crime—reduced trust but would not have long-lasting effects in the absence of broader structural changes.

3. The structural changes that best explain the long-term decline in trust include: value changes in attitudes toward authority and social restraints in general; economic destabilization stemming from technological change and globalization; changes in the political process that weakened political parties and increased the perceived distance between elites and the public; and a more consistent negative stance by the press toward government as well as other key institutions.[4]

No systematic evidence shows that younger Americans are more (or less) likely to trust government than are older Americans. In some respects, however, their attitudes toward government are more favorable than that of other age cohorts. For example, eighteen-to-twenty-five-year-olds are least likely to see government as inefficient and wasteful, or to believe that the federal government controls too much of Americans' daily lives (CIRCLE, 2002a).[5] If these youthful attitudes persist over time, they could provide a basis for renewed government activism in areas of national need such as health care.

Trust in Other Key Institutions

Governmental institutions in the United States were hardly alone in experiencing declining public trust during the past generation. Other major institutions to suffer that fate include labor, the legal profession, educational institutions, the media, and even organized religion. Confidence in business and corporations, which increased during the second half of the 1990s, has collapsed in the wake of recent highly publicized financial scandals. Only the police and the armed forces have managed to gain increased trust during this period.[6]

Trust in Other People

Americans' trust in one another has declined during the past generation, although less sharply than trust in government. From a high of 54 percent in the early 1960s, trust declined to only 34 percent in the early 1990s, where it remained, with minor oscillations, for the remainder of the decade. Unlike trust in government, evidence suggests that young people are significantly less likely to trust others than do older citizens.[7] As recently as 1975, high school students trusted other people at the same rate as adults did; by the late 1990s, a gap of nearly 15 points had opened up between high school students and other adults. Indeed, most, if not all, of the overall decline in social trust since the 1960s can be explained by the changing composition of the population. Older Americans are no less trusting than they were thirty years ago, but younger, less trusting Americans make up a larger and larger share of the population (Putnam, 2000).

No consensus exists among scholars concerning the causes of diminished trust in other people. The most plausible hypotheses include: the sharp increase in rates of crime and violence between the mid-1960s and the early 1990s; the disruption of family stability, especially through soaring rates of divorce; and immigration, which significantly increased the diversity of the U.S. population. Because these factors tended to affect young people disproportionately, they may explain why young people are now less likely to trust others.

In the wake of September 11, 2001, there were increases in trust in government (at all levels), in other institutions, and in other people. Civic behavior changed much less than civic attitudes, however, and recent evidence suggests that trust is declining toward pre–September 11 levels.

Other Key Attitudes

The past thirty years have seen a gradual shift toward materialism. Nowhere has that change been sharper than among young adults. In the mid-1960s, nearly 90 percent of college students believed that it was very important to develop a meaningful philosophy of life, versus about 40 percent who said that it was important to become well-off financially. By the beginning of the twenty-first century these sentiments had been reversed: 73 percent of college students said it was important to become well-off, versus only 42 percent who felt that way about developing a meaningful philosophy of life.[8] Not surprisingly, this trend has led to differences among age cohorts: toward the end of the 1990s, young adults reported significantly higher interest in money and self-fulfillment than other Americans, as well as much lower levels of patriotism.[9] (Here as elsewhere, it remains to be seen whether the changes produced by the events of September 11 will be temporary or long lasting).

Other important attitudinal shifts include: increased racial, ethnic, religious, and gender tolerance; and the increased value placed on unfettered individual choice as the central norm of U.S. social life (Putnam, 2000; Wolfe, 1998; Yankelovich, 1994).

Interest in Public Affairs

Over the past generation, Americans' interest in public affairs has steadily declined, by roughly one-fifth, with occasional spikes during unusual events (Putnam 2000). Key measures of declining interest include: reading about public affairs in newspapers; watching national television news; discussing politics; and the belief that it is important to keep up-to-date with political developments.

This decline has been especially pronounced among young people. In the mid-1960s, 60 percent said that they thought it was important to keep up with politics; by 2002, that figure had declined to less than 20 percent. In contrast, the decline in interest in public affairs for adults fifty years or over was smaller, though pronounced; in the mid-1960s, 62 percent said that keeping up with public affairs was important; in 2002 42 percent felt the same way. Every other measure of political interest fell by at least one-half during that period for young people.[10]

Party Affiliation and Ideology

Forty years ago, Americans who identified themselves as Democrats considerably outnumbered those who labeled themselves Republicans; relatively few regarded themselves as "independent"; and self-identified "liberals" outnumbered "conservatives." In the ensuing forty years, party identification tended to become more equal, the percentage of political independents increased, and self-identified conservatives increased to match (by some measures, exceed) liberals.

These trends have been especially pronounced among young adults. In 1972, college freshmen who regarded themselves as "liberal or far left" outnumbered those who identified as "conservative or far right" by 41 percent to 16 percent. By the mid-1990s, at the height of the electoral revolt against the Clinton administration, the liberal/far-left group fell to 25 percent, while the conservative/far-right rose to near-parity (24 percent). Even today, with the conservative tide ebbing from its high-water mark, only 28 percent of college freshmen think of themselves as liberal/far left, versus 21 percent for conservative/far right. (Interestingly, a gender gap has opened up during this period;

unlike thirty years ago, young college women are now more likely to think of themselves as liberals than are young college men [CIRCLE, 2002b].) A recent comprehensive survey of young adults shows a three-way split: 30 percent call themselves Democrats, 28 percent Republicans, and 27 percent independents. Similarly, 32 percent think of themselves as liberal, 23 percent conservative, and 30 percent moderate.[11]

Among adults fifty years and older the movement toward conservatism has not been as pronounced as that among young people. In 1960, of adults fifty years and older, 46 percent identified themselves as Democrats, 19 percent as independents, and 35 percent as Republicans. By 2002, 39 percent of these adults identified themselves as Democrats, 32 percent independents, and 29 percent as Republicans in 2002. Similarly, the ideological identification of mature adults only changed slightly. In 1972, 19 percent of mature adults identified themselves as liberals, 39 percent as moderates, and 42 percent as conservatives. In 2002, among mature adults, 26 percent identified as liberals, 29 percent as moderates, and 45 percent as conservatives.[12]

Political Knowledge

Americans today know roughly as much about political institutions and events as they did fifty years ago. This stability is remarkable, given that education tends to increase political knowledge and that the median amount of formal education has risen by four years during the past half century. Today's college graduates know no more than high school graduates did fifty years ago, and today's high school graduates are no more knowledgeable than were the high school dropouts of the past.[13]

Equally disturbing is the developing generation gap in political knowledge. From the 1940s through the mid-1970s, young people were at least as well-informed as were older Americans. Starting with the baby boomers and accelerating with their children, this pattern has shifted drastically. As Robert Putnam summarizes, "Today's under-thirties pay less attention to the news and know less about current events than their elders do today or than people their age did two or three decades ago" (Putnam 2000, p. 36). Here, as elsewhere, the events of September 11, 2001, evoked an increased interest in political events among all Americans, and especially younger Americans.

However, current indications show that this surge represents a tempo-rary "spike" rather than a sustained shift toward interest in politics and current events.

CIVIC BEHAVIOR

Voting

A central indicator of civic behavior is the willingness of citizens to go to the polls on Election Day. Remarkably, there is no generally accepted method for measuring turnout in the United States; every existing method is significantly flawed.[14] Nonetheless, it is possible to examine broad trends over time with confidence.

For much of the twentieth century, voting rates in the United States were well below those of other democracies. Substantial variations occurred within that period, however: overall participation rose to a post–World War II peak in the early 1960s and declined significantly thereafter. Between the mid-1960s and the early 1970s, turnout dropped by about ten percentage points; it has declined much more slowly since then, by about four percentage points.

Recent scholarship has sought to explain this decline. The most persuasive attempt focuses on three factors—resources, interest, and mobilization. According to this thesis, increasing economic inequal-ity has deprived large numbers of poor and undereducated Americans of the resources they need to participate, while the decline of Ameri-can political parties as grassroots organizations has diminished voter mobilization. Meanwhile, events have tended to depress interest in politics among Americans born after the civic-minded Depression/World War II generation. Although it has long been the case that vot-ing (and other forms of political activity) tends to increase with age, careful analysis suggests that in recent decades differences among generations have become more important in explaining voting behav-ior (Schlozman, Verba, & Brady, 1999).

For nearly a century after the Civil War, African Americans were systematically denied the right to vote. With the great legal and con-stitutional changes of the 1960s, this began to change. Today, Afri-can-American voting rates are close to those of white Americans, with the rates of young African Americans surpassing those of young white Americans.[15] (Indeed, once education is taken into account, they are somewhat higher.)

Hispanics are the most rapidly growing sector of the U.S. electorate. For various reasons, however, their electoral participation has not reflected their increasing weight in the population. On average, Hispanics are younger, poorer, and less educated than other population groups, factors that depress turnout among voters generally. In addition, substantial numbers of Hispanics are not yet citizens and are therefore ineligible to vote in most jurisdictions. Still, the voting rate among Hispanics who are U.S. citizens remains lower than that of other groups in the electorate.[16]

This may now be changing, however. Many Hispanics interpreted anti-immigrant legislation enacted in California in the mid-1990s as hostile to their ethnic group. Changes in federal welfare legislation reinforced that view. The result has been highly visible Hispanic voter mobilization, especially in large cities where Hispanics now hold the balance of political power and where promising Hispanic candidates for mayor and city council are coming forward.

An important change occurred in 1971, when for the first time Americans as young as eighteen years old were allowed to vote. At first, they participated in substantial numbers: in the presidential election of 1972, 53 percent of eligible voters aged eighteen to twenty-five cast ballots. Over the next thirty years, the rate of participation in that age group fell sharply; by the 2000 presidential election, only 37 percent of young Americans bothered to vote, a decline of roughly one-third. Similar trends are apparent for congressional elections held during nonpresidential election years. In 1974, 26 percent of Americans aged eighteen to twenty-five voted for congressional candidates; in 1998, only 19 percent cast their ballots—again, a decline of roughly one-third. In contrast, there has been little change in the voter turnout rates of mature adults; in 1972 70 percent of eligible mature adults voted and in 2000 69 percent voted. For midterm elections, in 1974, 57 percent of eligible mature adults voted, while in 1998 60 percent voted (Levi & Lopez, 2002).

The level of education affects voter participation throughout the U.S. population, but its effect on younger voters is especially pronounced. In the presidential election of 2000, only 21 percent of young Americans with less than a high school education voted, as compared to 69 percent of college graduates (Levi & Lopez, 2002). In contrast, among mature adults in 2000, 50 percent of high school dropouts voted while 84 percent of those with a college degree voted, a smaller gap than among young people. Furthermore, in the overall population, 86 percent of college graduates voted, but so did 47 percent of high school dropouts.

Other Forms of Participation in Official Politics

Americans participate in politics in many others forms other than voting—for example, writing to their elected representative, signing petitions, and attending rallies. The conventional wisdom is that while Americans are below average in voting, they are very active by international standards in other aspects of political participation. This belief is less true than it used to be. Between 1973 and 1994, the Roper organization conducted an annual survey of political participation, which examined trends in twelve different activities. During those two decades, every one of the indicators of participation declined significantly. The decline was especially steep (between 34 and 42 percent) for those activities that required working with others in public settings. (By contrast, the more solitary political activities—writing one's congressman or senator, signing a petition, writing a letter to the editor of a newspaper—experienced smaller declines.) Overall, there was a decrease of 25 percent in the share of Americans who participated in at least one of the twelve activities during the prior year.[17]

Like voting, participation in these other political activities is strongly influenced by wealth, education, and social position. Participation increases steadily as income rises, and citizens in the top income quintile are roughly five times as likely to engage in a political activity as are those in the bottom quintile (Brady, Schlozman, Verba, & Elms, 2002). (This ratio has fluctuated between four and seven over the past quarter century, with a mean of roughly five [Brady et al., 2002].)

Political participation is also affected by age. Young people are least likely to participate, but engagement tends to rise steadily through middle age before falling again among the elderly. In addition, today's Americans at every age level are less likely to participate than were Americans of comparable ages in previous generations (Putnam, 2000).

Putnam's analysis shows that this process of declining participation has contributed to the polarization of American politics. Individuals who identify themselves as moderate, centrist, or middle-of-the-road have been disproportionately likely to drop out of politics, while those who are more ideologically extreme have tended to remain active. This helps explain an apparent paradox: while an increasing fraction of the U.S. electorate identifies itself as moderate (rather than very liberal or very conservative), fewer and fewer elected representatives are moderates (Putnam, 2000). Political parties have learned that ideologically committed voters are more likely to vote, donate money, and participate in grassroots organizing, so campaigns are increasingly aimed at mobilizing this intense base of support, which further alienates moderates, and so forth, in a vicious circle.

Voluntary Organizations

Since the publication of Tocqueville's *Democracy in America,* Americans have seen themselves (and have been seen by others) as unusually likely to address social and political problems by forming voluntary organizations. Although there is much truth to this view, recent scholarship has pointed to some disturbing trends. Since 1995, Robert Putnam has been arguing that the fabric of American civil society has been fraying. With the publication of *Bowling Alone,* even the skeptics were forced to concede that there was substantial evidence of decline.

Putnam was able to show, for example, that membership in major national organizations has declined, as has active participation in local clubs and groups. Union membership has fallen from almost 35 percent of the workforce to less than 15 percent. Even church attendance appears to have fallen off, though less steeply than participation in secular groups. In the main, organizations that have grown in the past generation have tended to be "checkbook" organizations, which use direct mail to raise funds for the support of national headquarters and professional advocacy rather than face-to-face activities among local citizens (Putnam, 2000).

One might suppose that participation in civil society would be less influenced by income and status than is participation in official politics. But in fact, we observe much the same influence of socioeonomic standing in civil society. Once again, there is a linear relation between social position and group membership; those at the top are three times as likely to participate as are those at the bottom (Brady et al., 2002).

The major exception to this generalization is religion. No relation exists between social position and attending religious services or meetings. Individuals of all income levels are equally likely to participate, and this equality has persisted virtually unchanged over the past thirty years (Brady et al., 2002). The mobilization of religious Americans over the past generation represents one of the few tendencies toward political and civil equalization during this period.

Giving and Volunteering

Closely related to membership in civic organizations are the activities of giving (charitable contributions) and volunteering in neighborhoods and communities. Here trends are mixed. Charitable contributions peaked at about 2.2 percent of national income in the mid-1960s and have fallen fairly steadily ever since, to about 1.6 percent today.[18] (Measured in real dollars per capita, charitable giving rose during this period, reflecting the large increase in per capita income. However, most scholars believe that it is more meaningful to measure contributions in relation to individual, family, or national income.)

Volunteering is the principal exception to the general pattern of weakening civic involvement. Over the past twenty-five years, volunteering by the average American has risen from six times per year to nearly eight times. Much of this increase has occurred among older Americans, who are enjoying longer, healthier, more prosperous retirements than ever before. (Volunteering is up a remarkable 140 percent among Americans over the age of seventy-five.) We also observe significant increases among college students and young adults. Only among Americans age thirty to fifty has volunteering stagnated or declined since 1975 (Putnam, 2000).

The increase in volunteering among young people is contested. Anecdotal evidence suggests that more and more young people are being required to volunteer by their schools as a condition of high school graduation, or by colleges and universities as a condition of admission. When questioned, however, young people deny that these requirements are a major factor. Rather, they claim they volunteer because someone asked, because it makes them feel good, or because they want to make a difference. Nearly a quarter of all young Americans see volunteering as an alternative to participation in a political system they regard as remote, unresponsive, and beholden to special interests.[19]

Social Movements

Social movements would seem to be a conspicuous exception to the broad pattern of declining civic engagement summarized in this chapter. After all, since the early 1960s U.S. society has been transformed by movements for civil rights, feminism, environmentalism, gay and lesbian rights, and many others. Many activists believe that the past forty years have been a golden age for social movements.

The evidence suggests, however, that few of these movements have achieved sustained mass mobilization. Today, most consist of small cadres of professional advocates sustained by large numbers of citizens whose main mode of participation is writing checks. It is doubtful whether this mode of civic engagement builds social capital, especially at the local and community level (Putnam, 2000).

CONCLUSION

On balance, the evidence presented in this chapter supports the conclusion that civic life in the United States is weaker overall than it was a few decades ago. The World War II generation, which contributed so much to the vitality of U.S. politics and civil society, is dying off. The oldest baby boomers, born in 1946, are now close to sixty years old and within striking distance of retirement. Indeed, by the time this chapter is published, half of all boomers will have joined the ranks of adults aged fifty or older. It remains to be seen whether this new generation of mature adults will contribute as much as their parents did to their country's civic life.

NOTES

1. For the historical record, see Ladd & Bowman (1998), p. 15.
2. See especially Rahn (1998, 1999).
3. For the best study of recent developments, see Kohut (1998).

4. See Nye, Zelikow, & King (1997), pp. 268-276.
5. See Keeter, Zukin, Andolina, & Jenkins, 2002, p. 39.
6. See Ladd & Bowman (1998), Chapter 6.
7. See Rahn (1998).
8. See CIRCLE (2002b), p. 3.
9. See Rahn (1999).
10. See CIRCLE (2002b), p. 5; also Bennett (1997). The 2002 figures are based on authors' tabulations from the American National Election Study.
11. See Lake Snell Perry & Associates/The Tarrance Group, Inc. (2002).
12. All figures based on authors' tabulations from the American National Election Study, 1960, 1972, and 2002.
13. For all this and much more, see especially Delli Carpini & Keeter (1996).
14. For a discussion of these difficulties, see Lopez (2002).
15. See Lopez (2003b), p. 2.
16. See Lopez (2003a), pp. 2-3.
17. This survey is summarized in Putnam (2000), p. 45.
18. This trend is summarized in Putnam (2000), p. 124. Figure 31 on that page also shows that the mid-1960s peak represents a remarkable increase from the roughly 1.5 percent characteristic of the 1930s. This raises the question whether the Depression/World War II generation should be regarded as an aspirational norm or rather an unusual exception to typical social patterns.
19. See Lake Snell Perry & Associates/The Tarrance Group, Inc. (2002), pp. 10-13, 20.

REFERENCES

Bennett, S.E. (1997). Why young Americans hate politics, and what we should do about it. *PS: Political Science & Politics,* March: 47-53.

Brady, H.E., Schlozman, K.L., Verba, S., & Elms, L. (2002). Who bowls? The (un)changing stratification of participation. In B. Narrande and C. Wilcox (Eds.), *Understanding public opinion* (2nd ed.). Washington, DC: CQ Press.

Center for Information and Research on Civic Learning and Engagement (CIRCLE). (2002a, January 9). Youth civic engagement after 9/11. CIRCLE and the Pew Center for the People and the Press. College Park, MD: CIRCLE.

Center for Information and Research on Civic Learning and Engagement (CIRCLE). (2002b, January 9). Youth civic engagement: Basic facts and trends. College Park, MD: CIRCLE.

Delli Carpini, M.X. & Keeter, S. (1996). *What Americans know about politics and why it matters.* New Haven, CT: Yale University Press.

Keeter, S., Zukin, C., Andolina, M., & Jenkins, K. (September 2002). *The civic and political health of the nation: A generational portrait.* College Park, MD: CIRCLE.

Kohut, A. (1998). *Deconstructing distrust: How Americans view government.* Washington, DC: Pew Research Center for the People and the Press.

Ladd, E.C. & Bowman, K.H. (1998). *What's wrong: A survey of American satisfaction and complaint.* Washington, DC: The AEI Press.

Lake Snell Perry & Associates/The Tarrance Group, Inc. (March 2002). Short-term impacts, long-term opportunities: The political and civic engagement of young adults in America. Analysis and report for the Center for Information and Research on Civic Learning and Engagement (CIRCLE). College Park, MD: CIRCLE.

Levi, P. & Lopez, M.H. (September 2002). *Youth voter turnout has declined, by any measure.* College Park, MD: CIRCLE.

Lopez, M.H. (2003a). Electoral engagement among Latinos. *Latino Research at Notre Dame,* 1(2): 2-3.

Lopez, M.H. (2003b). Electoral engagement among Latino youth. College Park, MD: CIRCLE.

Nye, J.S. Jr., Zelikow, P.D., & King, D.C. (1997). *Why people don't trust government.* Cambridge, MA: Harvard University Press.

Pew Research Center. (2002). Americans struggle with religion's role at home and abroad. Available online at: http://people-press.org/reports/print.php3?ReportID=150.

Post-Modernity Project. (1966). *The state of disunion.* Charlottesville, VA: University of Virginia.

Putnam, R.D. (2000). *Bowling alone: The collapse and revival of American community.* New York: Simon & Schuster.

Rahn, W. (1998). Generations and American national identity: A data essay. Prepared for presentation at the Communication in the Future of Democracy Workshop, Annenberg Center, Washington, DC, May 8-9.

Rahn, W. (1999). Americans' engagement with and commitment to the political system: A generational portrait. Prepared for presentation at the COSSA Congressional Briefing, Washington, DC, July 16.

Schlozman, K.L., Verba, S., & Brady, H.E. (1999). Civic participation and the equality problem. In T. Skocpol and M.P. Fiorina (Eds.), *Civic engagement and American democracy.* Washington, DC: Brookings/Russell Sage.

Wolfe, A. (1998). *One nation, after all.* New York: Viking.

Yankelovich, D. (1994). How changes in the economy are reshaping American values. In H.J. Aaron, T.E. Mann, & T.Taylor (Eds.), *Values and public policy.* Washington, DC: Brookings.

Zill, N. (2002). Civics lessens: Youth and the future of democracy. *Public Perspective,* January/February: 28.

Chapter 2

Social Capital and Civic Engagement of Individuals Over Age Fifty in the United States

Thomas H. Sander
with Robert D. Putnam

A visual inspection of civic groups across the country shows the dominance of elderly Americans, whether on nonprofit boards, in houses of worship, in neighborhood associations, etc.[1] But is this immemorial truth? Have elderly Americans always been the backbone of our civic life and will this trend continue? One can never ascertain this from any fixed point in time, but we can draw insights from examining surveys done over time. First, however, I take a bit of a diversion to discuss why civic engagement (and social capital more specifically) is important and what is happening to those trends overall.

Insightful chroniclers of American life dating back to de Tocqueville realized that civic engagement was a core component of America's strength. It was through voluntary associations that citizens discussed, experimented, and took action to improve American life, made informed political choices, and held government accountable.

Social capital, the social networks and the values, norms, and understandings that arise along these networks and facilitate cooperation, is one way of capturing the value that de Tocqueville and others observed.[2] The volume of research on social capital, both in the United States and worldwide, has mushroomed over the last decade.[3] This research has covered topics as diverse as the use of social capital in common pool resources in the high Andes; the impact of social capital on solid waste disposal in Bangladesh; how social capital relates to Russian mortality rates; or the role of familial social capital in Appalachian youth attainment. In addition, the literature as a whole shows, far beyond the United States, how social capital plays a critical role in ensuring safe streets, educated citizens, strong public health, economic growth, responsive government, and even the happiness of citizens.[4]

OVERALL TRENDS IN SOCIAL CAPITAL

If social capital is such a linchpin for American society, what has happened to its levels of social capital over the past decade? A full treatment of this would take hundreds of pages. In short, Americans have witnessed serious erosions in their stock of social capital in just one generation, whether one looks at informal social connections (getting together with neighbors, family dinners, entertaining friends, or picnics), political participation, philanthropy, engagement in voluntary associations (such as the PTA, Rotary, or 4-H), religious participation, or even general trust of others.[5] To put an order of magnitude around this decline, American[6] levels of social capital and civic engagement have probably fallen 25 to 30 percent over the past generation, a period in which average levels of education have skyrocketed, which should have fueled a dramatic *expansion* in levels of civic engagement.[7]

Although levels of social capital in America differ markedly by social class, size of city, state, education, etc., the declines in social capital have spared no sector of society with one exception. What Robert Putnam calls the "long civic generation"—those born between 1910 and 1940—and what Tom Brokaw refers to as the "greatest generation" are now, and have been throughout their entire lives, far more civic. In greater numbers than any other generation they read newspapers, give blood, vote, volunteer, etc. (This is obviously a broad generalization of the trends, and I give greater detail as follows.) Putnam (2000) believes that it is likely due to the "greatest generation" being spared the corrosive influence of television (since they came of age prior to its widespread dissemination) and the sense of civic solidarity, hard work, and selflessness that developed of necessity from living through two World Wars and the Great Depression.[8]

The coupling of these trends—clear generational differences in levels of social capital and the decline in social capital over the past generation—mean that the civic declines witnessed in America are less about individuals changing their civic attitudes and habits and more about generational replacement (i.e., American society becoming composed of generations that are on average less civic than earlier generations). This type of change is harder to overcome, since it is less about individuals resuming prior civic habits, and more about "teaching old dogs new civic tricks" (or habits at least). Putnam has used the analogy of trying to walk up a down-escalator: as older cohorts die off, their replacement with younger, less-civic cohorts automatically depresses average levels of civic engagement. Individuals will have to work to overcome this downward momentum.

LIFE CYCLE VERSUS GENERATIONAL TRENDS

Before proceeding, I should backtrack a bit to unpack the previous conclusion. At any one point in time one can't discern life-cycle patterns (how much of an activity people do at one age than another) from generational patterns (people born between two specific birth years always do more or less of this).

For example, attendance at pop/rock concerts is almost purely life-cycle related. If one compares the ages of rock-concert goers in 1975 with those in 1998 (see Figure 2.1) you find that the young have always attended more than middle-aged or senior Americans. If it were purely generational, you would expect a big increase between 1975 and 1998 in middle-aged Americans attending rock concerts (since the rock-concert-going habits they developed as kids would have stuck

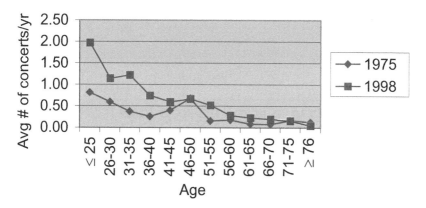

FIGURE 2.1. Rock concert attendance continues to be a young persons' activity.

with them all their lives). But instead, while everyone attends rock concerts somewhat more than in 1975, the biggest increases have been among the youngest generation and, if anything, have made rock-concert activity even more of a young person's sport.

Most activities, however, are a combination of life-cycle and generational patterns. For example, if one looks at how frequently Americans jog (see Figure 2.2) one finds that the young jog more frequently than any other age group, but that in 1975 there was a spurt in seniors jogging. This is likely generational. If it were a life-cycle phenomenon we would expect to see a similar experience in 1998 among seniors. It is possible that there were high levels of injury among seventy-one- to seventy-five-year-olds jogging in 1975 and doctors now discourage seniors from jogging or that they've simply moved on to yoga or swimming. Thus, jogging generally exhibits a life-cycle pattern (where young do it more) but with some generational component, for example, among the folks born between 1900 and 1904.

As Robert Putnam (2000) points out in *Bowling Alone* the distinction as to whether some activity is primarily life cycle or generational has stark implications for the patterns over time. In the case of purely life-cycle phenomena, society as a whole does not change,[9] even though individuals change their patterns from year to year as they age through the life cycle, because these individual changes cancel out at the aggregate level. Generational activities have the reverse dynamic: individuals don't change but society does. If, as is true, Americans born after 1945 are more racially tolerant,[10] then even if individual

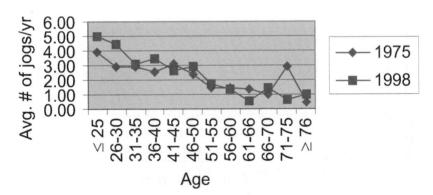

FIGURE 2.2. Jogging is a young persons' sport, with the exception of seniors in 1975.

Americans do not become any more racially tolerant over time, America as a whole will, as the less-tolerant Americans born pre-1945 die off over time and are replaced by more tolerant younger groups of Americans.

Behaviors that are driven by life cycle usually are attributable to one of the following: energy levels and health; family demands or family activities that connect individuals into communities; available time; or stage of career or skill and knowledge levels. Thus, involvement in the PTA centers around ages when people are typically child-rearing. On the other hand, "X-treme" skiers tend to be younger because the energy levels and fearlessness required are more apt to be found among younger Americans.

Knowing whether an activity is generational or life cycle is also critically important for predicting the future. For example, a central question that gets asked by groups such as the AARP (American Association of Retired Persons) or other nonprofit groups is how much boomers will volunteer when they retire. I will return to this question at the end.

A snapshot of who volunteered in America (see Figure 2.3) in 2000 shows older Americans volunteering almost as frequently as middle-aged Americans.[11] The temptation is to assume that the shape of this curve is fixed; if this is true, as the baby boomer demographic bulge nears retirement, we'll see an explosion of volunteering as 77 million Americans move into this high-volunteering phase of life.

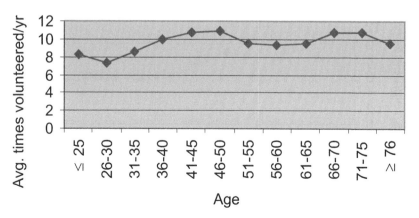

FIGURE 2.3. Volunteering, by age cohort, according to the 2000 Social Capital Benchmark Survey.

On the other hand, if retirement age is always associated with high rates of volunteering (a life-cycle phenomenon) than this should have been the case back in 1975. Figure 2.4 shows this wasn't nearly as true. Back in 1975, we also see the thirty- to forty-year-olds volunteering heavily (since life-cycle-driven family obligations, and child and work attachments engaged them in social networks that led them into volunteering). In 1975, we see only a modest concentration among volunteering for those over age seventy-five and we do not see any significant volunteering rate among Americans fifty-six to seventy-five years of age.

The juxtaposition of these two graphs (Figures 2.3 and 2.4) suggests that the boom among volunteering in senior Americans stems from the fact that the long civic generation, characterized by enormous civic motivation, is now postretirement and has a lot more time to volunteer and that the boomers (who have never been an especially strong volunteering cohort) will have to suddenly develop new stripes if they are going to volunteer in record numbers as they retire.

GENERATIONAL TRENDS
BEYOND VOLUNTEERING

Comparing the same question over time enables one to sort out generational patterns from life-cycle patterns.[12] By conducting surveys at multiple points in time,[13] one can analyze results by the birth

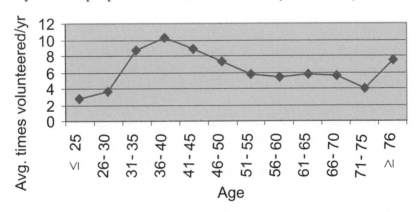

FIGURE 2.4. Volunteering, by age cohort (in 1975), according to DDB Lifestyles data.

year of respondent and see whether Americans born between 1940 and 1950 (for example) consistently do more or less of an activity regardless of the year in which the survey was administered. One can also look at two points of time and see whether the life-cycle curve has changed or not (as we did in the previous rock concert example). Observing charts of various civic activities tracked against the year of respondents' births show the broad declines—that, in general, Americans born early in the twentieth century are more engaged than the generations which came later (see Figure 2.5).

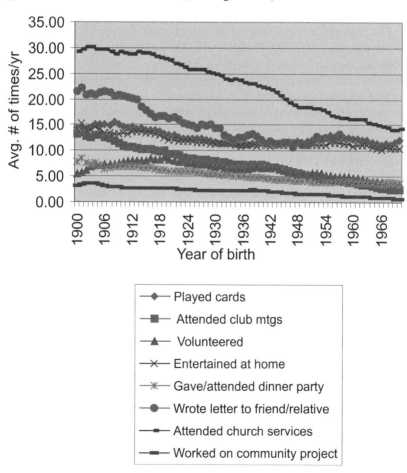

FIGURE 2.5. Civic activities are declining by generation.

One of the most thorough surveys on social capital, the Social Capital Community Benchmark Survey (SCCBS 2002), was conducted at a simple point in time: 2000. We'll look at age trends in the SCCBS, but, where the questions were similar, compare them to the DDB Lifestyles (1997, 1998) and Roper surveys (Roper Center, 1973-1994) to get a sense of whether the SCCBS results have held up over time.

SOCIAL CAPITAL COMMUNITY BENCHMARK SURVEY

The Social Capital Community Benchmark Survey was conducted in the summer of 2000. Roughly 27,000 Americans across 41 communities, and a national sample of 3,000 Americans, were polled on their levels of social capital.[14] Questions asked everything from informal social connections, to involvement in formal voluntary associations, to levels of trust of various groups, to the diversity of individuals' social ties. The communities surveyed spanned all parts of the country and encompassed huge cities (such as Chicago or Los Angeles) and tiny communities such as Bismarck, North Dakota, or the Kanawha Valley, West Virginia.[15]

In cases where the same question was asked, the results described are consistent with the DDB Lifestyles survey or Roper surveys and hold up when controlling for income, years of education, self-reported health, working status, gender, and marital status. (If not, this is noted in the footnotes or text.)

A clear majority of civic variables in 2000 show an *increase with age:* specifically *politics*[16] (voting, being registered to vote, political knowledge, attending rallies or political meetings, reading the paper, and political interest), *religiosity* (religious membership, attendance, religious philanthropy),[17] *all forms of trust* (trust of others, trust of shopkeepers, cops, co-religionists, media, etc., and even trust of other racial groups), *formal civic engagement* (being officers of groups, the number of groups with which the respondent was involved), and personal friendships with people who the respondent considered to be a community leader. This is fully consistent with the long civic generation, as current seniors have been especially political and religious all their lives. The high levels of trust asserted by older Americans are probably a function of the higher trustworthiness exhibited by their friends. This could stem from values imparted by the Great Depression and two world wars, or from the fact that through their stronger political and religious social networks, seniors would pay a higher cost for being untrustworthy than younger Americans who are living relatively more anonymous lives.

Relatively fewer variables in 2000 are higher for ages eighteen to twenty-four and then decrease with age. For example, many forms of *informal social engagement* (inviting friends over to your home,[18] hanging out with friends, socializing with work colleagues, participating in team sports, frequency of visiting relatives [which exhibited a more *mild relationship*], participating in groups, the arts, attending parades), participating in a march, or giving blood; many forms of *bridging relationships* (this is explained later but includes having personal friends who are gay, white,[19] black, Hispanic, or Asian, or having friends of different races over to your home).

Most of the civic do-gooding variables other than political electoral participation, religion, and trust, showed an inverted U-shape function (∩) where people do more of these activities in the middle-years (with different peaks depending on the different variables) and do less of this activity in the younger and older age cohorts. The seven civic do-gooding variables that exhibit a ∩ *shape with respect to age* are signing a petition, taking local action for social or political reform, engaging in a community project, working with immediate neighbors to fix or improve something, perceived impact in making community a better place, likelihood of cooperating to save water or electricity if there was a dire shortage, or attending a public meeting at which town or local affairs are discussed.

Despite the fact that younger cohorts had more education than the eldest cohorts, if one controls simultaneously for income, years of education, self-reported health, work status, and marital status, the relationship of virtually all these variables to age stays the same.

BRIDGING AND TOLERANCE

As the United States and most industrialized countries become increasingly racially and culturally diverse,[20] one very important civic attribute is the extent to which individuals and communities bridge social divides. (By bridging social divides, I mean social relationships that cross various societal cleavages, such as race, social class, religion, etc. In contrast to a bridging social tie, a bonding social tie links an individual with another who is like him or her along some dimension. In society, any given social tie could be bonding along one dimension and bridging along another. For example, a relationship between an African-American PhD and an African-American high school dropout would be bridging with respect to education [and probably social class] and bonding with respect to race.) We know that bonding social ties are much easier to create and much more prevalent than bridging social ties; this is not a new finding, it's captured in the proverb "birds of a feather flock together" that dates back to biblical times (according to some).

What do the SCCBS data tell us about bridging?[21] Younger respondents are more likely to have *racially* bridging friendships or to have gay friends (or at least know that their friends are gay). Specifically, younger respondents are more likely to have personal friends of a different race that are Asian, black, or Hispanic[22] or visit with friends of a different race, more likely to participate in groups that have racial bridging, and are more tolerant of interracial marriage. Although it is true that younger respondents are more likely to live in slightly more racially diverse environments, these patterns don't disappear when one adjusts for this.[23]

Interestingly, younger Americans don't bridge more for all types of bridging. Older Americans appear to bridge more across religion, and are slightly more likely to bridge with respect to gender and education, and possibly slightly more across class. In addition, older nonwhites are more likely than younger nonwhites to have personal racial bridging friendships to whites.

The fact that older Americans are more religious accounts for much of why older Americans are more likely to have bridging ties across religious lines. These relationships hold up even adjusting for older Americans' increased religious attendance, religious membership, religious participation outside of services, and the importance older Americans attach to religion. It is possible that some of the differences between generations relate to older Americans being raised in an era in which religious ties held greater importance. For example, people who came of age in the 1950s frequently recall knowing the religion of every other boy and girl in their high school class, not out of idle curiosity, but because religious affiliation told you which boys were your competition for which girls in an era of religious endogamy. It is far rarer among Americans coming of age in the 1970s to have known the religious affiliation of their high school classmates since religious endogamy had largely eroded by that point. Thus some of the differences reported between different generations might stem from older Americans being more likely to know which of their friendships cross religious lines than younger Americans.[24]

Why do older nonwhite Americans have more cross-racial friendships with whites than younger Americans? This reflects a difference between white and nonwhite respondents in their levels of racially bridging relationships: for whites, the number of racially bridging relationships declines with age whereas for nonwhite Americans it slightly increases (see Figure 2.6). This trend occurs most for Hispanics, whereas 67 percent of Hispanics ages eighteen to twenty-four have personal friendships with non-Hispanic whites versus 82 to 90 percent of Hispanics ages sixty-one to seventy have such friendships, but even for blacks and Asians younger respondents are no more likely to have personal friends that cross racial lines than older respondents. This is indeed a puzzle, both sociologically and mathematically. If younger whites report higher levels of personal friendships with nonwhites (assuming, as is typically the case, that they are with similar-age nonwhites), then these higher levels should also show up for nonwhite younger respondents; but they do not.[25] For non-Hispanic whites, unlike respondents of color, tolerance and ra-

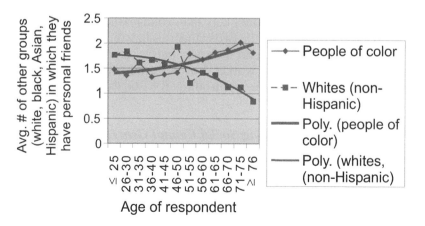

FIGURE 2.6. White racial bridges decline with age. Nonwhite bridging increases.

cially bridging relationships seem to go hand-in-hand: the youngest respondents are both the most tolerant and most likely to have racially bridging relationships. Scholars will need to explore more deeply the puzzle these SCCBS survey responses suggest: that younger whites have more racial bridges to nonwhites than older whites do, but younger nonwhites do not bridge more to whites than older nonwhites.[26]

Bridging by education and gender show less clear-cut trends. Uncontrolled for levels of education, marital status, etc., older Americans are a bit more likely to bridge across levels of education and about the same likelihood to be in groups that bridge across gender. Controlling for education, income, martial status, and work situation, older Americans (ages sixty-five and older) are statistically less likely to be in groups that are diverse with respect to gender than are forty-five- to fifty-five-year-olds, and younger cohorts ages eighteen to thirty-four are less likely to have bridging relationships across levels of education than forty-five- to fifty-five-year-olds.

Class Bridging

Although older respondents are less likely to bridge across race, there is no evidence that they are any less likely to bridge across class. Across some variables (e.g., having a personal friend that owns a vacation home or owns a business), older Americans are more likely to bridge across class, however, this may be a result of natural age biases in the wording of the question.[27] Consistent with this interpretation, older Americans are no more likely than young Americans (eighteen to thirty-four) to bridge in the two categories in which the wording of the question is least likely to have age biases: reporting a personal friendship with a manual worker[28] or personal friends to someone who has been on welfare, controlling for standard demographic factors.

Are Differences in Bridging Social Capital Generational or Life Cycle?

Research on the extent of bridging social ties is in its relative infancy and the SCCBS paved a lot of new ground in measuring bridging social capital. However, since the SCCBS is one point in time, we can't know for sure whether this increased bridging of younger respondents (by race and with gays) is generational (being born in the later third of the twentieth century) or life cycle (being young). (Since there are long-term trends showing that there have been generational changes in tolerance, it is reasonable to suppose that these higher bridging patterns are generational as well, but we'll only know this for sure over time.) If it proves to be generational, individuals won't change but society will (through generational replacement) and by 2020 or 2030 middle-aged Americans should be bridging a lot more than middle-aged Americans today. If instead it is life cycle (something about being young) these individuals will bridge less across race as they age, and this difference between young and old will remain.

Complicating this story about bridging social capital is the fact that almost all communities will become more diverse over time. Los Angeles, which is one of the most diverse communities of modern settlement, represents predicted average levels of diversity in the United States fifty to sixty years from now. Even if the inclination to bridge across racial lines doesn't exhibit generational patterns, our opportunity to forge bridging social capital will be much higher in 2030 than now. To pick up true patterns over time, we'd have to control for the opportunity to form bridging ties.

CONCLUSION

In this chapter, we've tried to lay out the evidence for how civic habits and patterns differ by generation. The long civic generation is buttressing political and religious engagement and trust among seniors. The civic differences among Americans today are mostly generational. Younger Americans are more likely to engage in most forms of informal social engagement (meeting with friends, family, and job colleagues). These age-related differences are, by contrast, largely life cycle. Thus, the former differences portend broader social changes, whereas the latter do not.

With the fast-approaching retirement of baby boomers, American society will be markedly affected by what civic patterns boomers exhibit as they retire. This will effect everything from the political potency of AARP (When they say "vote" or "call your congressperson" will boomers listen?) to the long-term viability of nonprofit groups and boards that depend on volunteer labor to the livelihood of specific churches and the public health of boomers as they retire.[29]

On this last point of health, one often hears about the impressive rise in longevity among Americans over the twentieth century.[30] It boosted life expectancy at birth roughly 30 years from 47.3 in 1900 to 77 years in 2000.[31] Most of this gain in life expectancy came originally from dramatic reductions in infant and child mortality in the first half of the twentieth century.[32] In the second half of the twentieth century, the gains to life expectancy came from gains among older Americans: life expectancy at age sixty-five rose about a third from 13.9 additional years in 1950 to 18.0 additional years in 2000. Medical experts, having effectively wiped out most infectious diseases and childhood mortality, focused on cardiovascular disease, cancer, and chronic conditions of the elderly. By 2000, gains to life expectancy slowed, despite aggressive investments in medical technology. The standard suspects for these slowing declines are obesity and especially resistant viral diseases; less explored alternative explanations are declines in social capital. Boomers face a threefold social capital penalty: (1) they have fewer friends than their parents,[33] (2) fewer children than their parents, and (3) are more likely to be single or divorced than their parents.[34] Fewer friends, fewer children, and fewer spouses all translate into shriveled social support networks—fewer people to bring one chicken soup when one is ill. Based on other research on the connections between social capital and health, boomers' weaker social capital should, along with obesity and viral diseases, likely result in weakened health prospects for the coming ranks of seniors.

A central challenge in getting boomers more involved is that religion has been a major engine for senior volunteering in the past and boomers are not an especially religious cohort. Moreover, boomers appear to be less involved than their parents and middle age is usually the peak for volunteering, so we may be at a high-water mark for volunteering unless we alter the normal shape of the curve.

More optimistically, some forces are rallying to try to change the shape of the curve. A recent conference convened at Harvard University focused on whether boomers will become civic as they retire and what might increase this likelihood. The conclusions are a bit bullish given the boomers' track record, but the report makes for very interesting reading.[35] Conference organizers voiced concern that we may need to reinvent volunteering and see how it can be tied into lifelong learning and engagement, provide boomers with a social circle through volunteering, think about how boomers who haven't provided for their own retirement can both "volunteer" and make ends meet, and make sure that organizations are positioned to use boomers effectively. Other groups such as Civic Ventures, Experience Corps or AmeriCorps/Senior Corps, or Elderhostel are also focused on seeing what institutions would encourage boomers to get more civically involved.

Given their large numbers, even modest changes in the boomers' trajectory could have dramatic consequences. All parents and grandparents should hope that these efforts succeed as they will directly shape how civically nutritious a culture and legacy our children and grandchildren will inherit.

NOTES

1. This chapter focuses on the United States because the U.S. data are strongest on this question; the relationship between age and social capital may or may not differ in other countries. *Democracies in Flux* (Putnam, 2000) demonstrated at least that the trends in social capital are not always parallel across the globe. In addition, the recent European Social Survey (2003) on immigration and social capital shows that the distribution of social capital across age groups looks very different in Europe, but there is no way without repeated surveys over time to separate out whether these differences are generational (and thus will not persist) or life cycle (and thus will persist) and whether there have always been these international differences or whether the differences are more recent.

2. Differences exist among scholars concerning the precise definition of social capital, but social capital researchers are coming to consensus around a "lean and mean" definition that focuses on the social networks and the values and norms that they engender. Most feel that trust and reciprocity probably shouldn't be included directly (but are close correlates that usually arise as a consequence). See for example the definition of social capital in *The Well-Being of Nations: The Role of Human and Social Capital* (OECD, 2001). Social capital, like any form of capital, is not monolithic. (Physical capital, for example, includes pencils and steam turbines, both useful for very different things.) More work needs to be done on dimensionalizing social capital, but a discussion of some of the likely dimensions can be found in *Democracies in Flux* (Putnam, 2000), at pp. 6-12.

3. There were two or fewer academic papers annually on social capital until the publication of *Making Democracy Work* (Putnam, Leornardi, & Raffaella, 1994) and *Bowling Alone* (Putnam, 2000); since then the number of papers mushroomed to sixty-one in 1997 and 292 in 2003. ISI Web of Science annual citation index available online at http://www.isinet.com/isi/products/citation/wos.

4. *Bowling Alone* contains a much fuller discussion on pp. 20-24 and pp. 287-366, with a stylized example at pp. 289-290. However, in sum, social capital is important because the social networks facilitate information flows; spread people's reputations more quickly (thus penalizing people who cheat or act in a purely self-interested way); facilitate recruiting others for collective action; obviate the need for negotiating the terms of every action to help another (since in social-capital-rich communities one is likely to be repaid later either directly by the beneficiary or by others in the community); and spare individuals from having to engage in defensive actions (counting change, locking the doors, writing defensive memos at work, etc.). See also Paul Seabright's (2004) *Company of Strangers,* which demonstrates that our ability to trust strangers without being taken advantage of is central to the progress and prosperity of humans in the modern age.

5. A full treatment of this decline can be found in *Bowling Alone* at pp. 183-286, along with a debunking of all the countertrends that Americans think offset the decline.

6. Less clarity exists about how universal these social capital declines have been. Ten scholars, led by Robert Putnam, in some ten industrialized countries worldwide investigated trends in social capital, and although the data are far from perfect, there are often echoes of the U.S. trends (or early shadows) in many of these countries. Even in the countries (like Sweden) that seem most immune from these trends thusfar, some see potential dark clouds on the horizon. For a fuller discussion of these global trends see *Democracies in Flux* (Putnam, 2000, note 1).

7. The best demographic predictor for levels of social capital and civic engagement is an individual's level of education.

8. The circumstances of the long civic generation can be contrasted against that of the boomers who, rather than facing unifying circumstances, saw their generation driven by polarizing debates about the Vietnam war, civil rights, environmentalism, etc.

9. This presumes a relatively even distribution of the population across age groups so that the flow of population into and out of age cohorts is relatively constant. Obviously, if there is a huge demographic bulge coming into or leaving a specific age bracket (say the teenage years) and if an activity is heavily concentrated among this age bracket (e.g., skateboarding, which is very common among teens) one would see macro changes in the percentage of Americans doing an activity or the frequency of that activity.

10. This increase in tolerance halted with the boomers (Americans born in the 1970s or 1980s are no more tolerant than Americans born in the 1940s or 1950s).

11. Americans in their thirties and forties are significantly more likely to volunteer one or more times a year, but since senior American volunteers that do volunteer do so much more frequently than other Americans, senior Americans as a group volunteer almost as often on average as thirty- to forty-year-olds.

12. I am fortunate to have been able to access datasets such as DDB Lifestyles or Roper that ask the same question over time. These datasets are explained more fully in *Bowling Alone* (Putnam, 2000) at pp. 420-424.

13. What social scientists refer to as repeated cross-sections.

14. Although the forty-one communities were not randomly selected (and exhibited significant variation from community to community) collectively, the 27,000 "local" respondents and 3,000 national respondents look almost identical across almost any measure of social capital (there is essentially nothing on which they differ by more than 1 to 2 percent). This is why all 30,000 respondents were analyzed, not

just the national sample, as it enables us more effectively to control for multiple variables simultaneously.

15. Fuller description of the methodology of the twenty-five minute RDD phone survey, questions asked, and the data can be found at www.ropercenter.uconn.edu/scc_bench.html.

16. AARP, as one organization, has exploited the fact that senior Americans are so much more likely to vote than any other age cohort. We need to accept that this is a description of how America looks today, and is not a prediction that senior Americans will continue to vote far more than other Americans.

17. Religious participation (outside of worship services) increases until about age sixty and then drops slightly.

18. In the DDB Lifestyles Survey, the closest variable to this, entertaining friends in your home, exhibited a U-shape function where both the youngest and oldest respondents did this the most (1997 and 1998 data). The DDB question wording about "entertaining friends in one's home" vs. "visiting with friends in your home or theirs" may have more of an adult ring to it and may thus explain the differential patterns.

19. Personal friendships with people of certain races are coded as "bridging" relationships only if the respondent is not that race. Therefore, for a personal friendship with someone that is white to be bridging, the respondent would have to be nonwhite.

20. For example, in the United States, "people of color" (Hispanics and nonwhites) rose from 24 percent of the population in 1990 to 31 percent in 2001 and is projected to be nearly a majority of the country's population by 2050. Source: 2002 U.S. Statistical Abstract, Tables 14 and 16; 2001 U.S. Statistical Abstract, Table 17 (U.S. Census Bureau, 2001, 2002). Although the levels of diversity are much higher in the United States the trends of increasing racial and ethnic diversity are true of virtually all the industrialized countries of the world.

21. Again, with a single point one can't know whether trends by age are life cycle, generational, or a mix.

22. Interestingly, interracial bridges to whites *increase* with age (if you control for percent of whites in county, income, education, health, employment status, and gender), although only three of six age brackets were significant. Suggests that older nonwhites are more likely to bridge to whites than younger nonwhites.

23. This analysis uses the percentage of the "out group" at the county level, so for example, if one were analyzing the likelihood of having a bridging tie to a Hispanic, this controls for the percentage of Hispanics at the county level. If one were analyzing bridging ties to blacks, this would control for the percentage of blacks at the county level.

24. I noted earlier how self-reported bridging across lines of sexual orientation might exhibit the opposite pattern with respect to age. At least some scholars believe that the percentage of Americans who are homosexual has not changed dramatically over the past fifty years, but certainly people are much more aware of their sexual orientation and many are more open about it. Thus, in the case of sexual orientation, it is the younger cohort that may have a better idea of which of their friends are gay than older Americans and thus the higher reported incidence of gay friends among younger Americans may be partially due to increased awareness.

25. Although the SCCBS obviously did not survey all Americans, with a sample size of 30,000 almost all sampling error should be eliminated.

26. If anything, given the relative sizes of these populations in society, one would expect the reverse. In most communities surveyed in the SCCBS, whites were more numerous than nonwhites; thus, if there were x number of personal friendships between whites and nonwhites in a community, one would expect a higher percentage of nonwhites than whites would report having such friendships and thus increases in bridging relationships between whites and nonwhites should be magnified in the nonwhite community.

27. The SCCBS has only four measures of class bridging (do you have a personal friend that is a manual worker, owns a vacation home, has been on welfare, or owns a business). Since the question asks about whether the *respondent* has a personal friend that is a vacation-home owner, etc., we would probably expect that for vacation home owners and business owners these will have age biases. If most friendships are to people roughly of the same age, younger cohorts may have friends whose *parents* own businesses or vacation homes but are less likely to count these parents as personal friends. Both having a personal friend who owns a vacation home and having a personal friend that owns a business show a positive correlation with age of 0.077 and 0.047, respectively; this relationship holds true in a regression controlling for the diversity (Herfindahl) at the census tract level.

28. Respondents under age eighteen might be less likely to know a manual worker, but the SCCBS survey was only asked of respondents age eighteen or older.

29. Boomers' health are likely to be at risk since levels of civic engagement and social capital Among Americans is probably the strongest predictor of immunity to illness and rapid recovery when individuals do get sick.

30. The rise has actually been slower than in some industrialized countries (see, for example, Oeppen and Vaupel, 2002, Figure 2; note the gap between U.S. life expectancy and leading longevity nation has risen from less than a year in 1950 to five years in 2000).

31. See Table 27 from CDC National Center for Health Statistics publication *Health United States 2003*. See also National Vital Statistics Reports (2002), Vol. 51, No. 3.

32. For example, 20 percent of children died before age 10 in 1900 and this was well under 10 percent by 1940. By 1960, mortality due to infectious disease had basically been eliminated and infant deaths were quite rare.

33. In the SCCBS for example, boomers, despite being in the prime of their life, were almost one-third more likely to have two or fewer close friends (18.3 percent of those from long civic generation versus 24.5 percent of boomers).

34. For example, in SCCBS, boomers were over 40 percent more likely to be divorced or separated than the long civic generation (18.4 percent of boomers versus 12.9 percent of those from long civic generation).

35. See Reinventing Aging: Baby Boomers and Civic Engagement, available online at: http://www.hsph.harvard.edu/chc/reinventingaging/Report.pdf.

REFERENCES

CDC National Center for Health Statistics. (2003). Health United States 2003. Available online at www.cdc.gov/nchs/data/hus/tables/2003/03hus027.pdf.

DDB Lifestyles Survey Data. (1997). New York: DDB Heedham Advertising.
DDB Lifestyles Survey Data. (1998). New York: DDB Heedham Advertising.
European Social Survey on Immigration and Social Capital. (2003). London: Centre for Comparative Social Surveys.
National Vital Statistics Reports. (2002). Vol. 51, No. 3, Table 11. Available online at www.cdc.gov/nchs/fastats/pdf/nvsr51_03t11.pdf.
Oeppen, Jim & Vaupel, James W. (2002). Broken limits to life expectancy. *Science, 296* (May): 1029-1031.
Organisation for Economic Co-operation and Development (OECD). (2001). *The well-being of nations: The role of human and social capital.* London: OECD Publishing.
Putnam, Robert D. (2000). *Bowling alone.* New York: Simon & Schuster.
Putnam, Robert D. (Ed.). (2000). *Democracies in flux.* New York: Oxford University Press.
Putnam, Robert D., Leonardi, Robert, & Nanetti, Raffaella Y. (1994). *Making democracy work.* Princeton, NJ: Princeton University Press.
Roper Center for Public Opinion Research. (1973-1994). Roper social and political trends data 1973-1994. Order no. US Roper 1994 Trends. Storrs, CT: University of Connecticut.
Seabright, Paul. (2004). *Company of strangers.* Princeton, NJ: Princeton University Press.
Social Capital Community Benchmark Survey (SCCBS). (2002). Saquaro Seminar, Harvard University.
United States Census Bureau. (2001). U.S. Statistical abstract, table 17. Washington, DC: Author.
United States Census Bureau. (2002). U.S. Statistical abstract, tables 14 and 16. Washington, DC: Author.

PART II:
NATIONAL SERVICE
AND THE FIFTY-PLUS POPULATION

Chapter 3

Civic Engagement and National Service: Results from Senior Corps Evaluations

Priyanthi Silva
Cynthia Thomas

INTRODUCTION TO SENIOR SERVICE AND VOLUNTEERISM

In the United States there has been a tradition of engagement by seniors in volunteer activities with a civic purpose. These activities include informal services provided to families and friends as well as services provided through community organizations. Volunteering has encompassed "work in some way to help others for no monetary pay" (National Council on Aging, 1981), and "not based on obligation" (Ellis & Noyes, 1990), as well as more formal and organized types of activity. Volunteering sometimes has been defined exclusively in the context of not-for-profit organizations.

Volunteer programs serve two major functions. They (1) allow people to spend their leisure time in productive activities, and (2) provide service organizations with experienced, reliable, and willing workers at no cost. Often, senior volunteers serve through local institutions such as churches, museums, libraries, schools, and nursing homes. Elderly persons volunteer in diverse areas such as education, health care, public safety, and the environment. They offer care to children, provide transportation, deliver meals, and care for frail elderly. The enriched experiences of the elderly can be a valuable resource to meet community needs. Volunteer opportunities have gradually changed and demand has increased for volunteers to be more involved with mentoring, tutoring, and organizing after-school programs (Scheibel, 1996). Similarly, there is an increasing demand for volunteers to help with long-term care services (Thompson & Wilson, 2001) and home health care (Kilpatrick & Danziger, 1996).

Rates of participation in volunteer activities have gradually increased among the elderly, although precise rates of increase are difficult to ascertain since definitions are inconsistent across studies. Fischer & Schaffer (1993) estimated that the percentage of older people who are volunteers ranged from 11 to 52 percent. Several studies have placed the proportion of older persons (those fifty-five years and older) actively engaged in volunteer activities at about 26 percent (Caro & Bass, 1995; Herzog, Kahn, Morgan, Jackson, & Antonucci, 1989). Studies indicate that over time, and across definitions, the number of older people volunteering has been increasing in recent years. In 1998, 43 percent of those age seventy-five and over reported volunteering, an increase of 9 percentage points in only three years according to the Independent Sector (1999).

Despite relatively high rates of participation, according to some studies, the actual number of hours spent on service by volunteers varies considerably. Most studies find that the majority of volunteers contribute, on average, very little time. In 1981, for example, an NCOA/Harris survey found that 69 percent of older volunteers served less than seven hours a week, and another 26 percent served up to thirty-five hours a week (NCOA, 1981). Herzog & House (1991) found that on average volunteers serve only a few hours a week.

Demographic factors seem to influence volunteering (Fischer & Schaffer, 1993). Typically, those with higher levels of education (beyond high school), more income, and higher occupational status are more likely to participate than their less-educated and less-affluent peers. Recent increases in volunteering have not been directly linked by research to increasingly higher levels of educational attainment and greater financial security of older adults although a connection between them is plausible. Women have been found to volunteer in higher proportions than men (Kim & Hong, 1998; Independent Sector, 1999).

Volunteering differs to some extent by race and ethnicity, but recent information on such race/ethnic breakdowns by age is scarce. In 1981, a Harris survey for NCOA found low rates of formal volunteering among all groups, but slightly higher rates for whites (24 percent) than for blacks or Hispanics (17 and 12 percent, respectively). The Independent Sector (1999) reported increases in volunteering among both Hispanics and blacks of 6 to 12 percentage points in just four years but did not present these findings by age group. According to Fischer and Schaffer (1993), most minority populations in the United States have strong volunteer systems based on a tradition of informal helping. Most volunteering activity within the black community has been informal (Height, Toya, Kamikawa, & Maldonado, 1981). Informal volunteering also is reported to be common among the Native American and Asian communities since serving people in the community is part of their traditions. If the definition of volunteering included both formal and informal activities, the proportion of volunteers and the range of volunteer activities among the minority communities would be greater.

Married people are reported to volunteer more than the unmarried among both younger adults and the elderly. Marriage is correlated with higher income, especially when both the husband and wife are employed (Independent Sector, 1988). Good health and psychological well-being both strongly influence volunteering (Fischer, Mueller, Cooper, & Chase, 1989; Ozawa & Morrow-Howell, 1988; Independent Sector, 1988; Hunter & Linn, 1981). Many of the characteristics associated with higher rates of participation, such as higher levels of income and education and good health are on the increase among the elderly. These changes lead to the possibility that the potential volunteer force may grow at an even greater rate than the overall rate of increase in the older population.

Studies have noted the association between early volunteering habits and continuity of volunteering later on (Dye, Goodman, Roth, & Jensen 1973). The baby boomer generation has had a particularly high rate of volunteering and it will be important to see if this interest continues into retirement. Even nonvolunteers show a greater willingness to take on assignments after they have spent a couple of years in leisurely retirement (Bradley, 2000).

People between thirty-five and fifty-four years old are more likely to volunteer than people in any other age group. An important fact associated with volunteers in this age group is that they tend to volunteer most often in programs associated with their children—schools, sports, and other activities (Boraas, 2003). If parents concentrate on programs that affect their children and families, then the current wave of baby boomers now entering retirement may be called upon to fill the gap in providing services to meet other community needs. However, the attractiveness and relevance of available volunteer opportunities will determine the extent to which older people volunteer.

Large national organizations such as AARP and the United Way and federal agencies such as the Corporation for National and Community Service offer volunteer opportunities to seniors. The Corporation for National and Community Service (CNCS), the federal domestic volunteer agency with jurisdiction over the three nationwide Senior Corps programs for older volunteers, has been examining alternatives for the future. In particular, it has been exploring how well prepared it is to meet current and upcoming community service needs, and how best to incorporate the retiring baby boomers into its programs. A study was undertaken in 2000-2001 to determine the status of Senior Corps programs, the Foster Grandparent Program (FGP), the Senior Companion Program (SCP), and the Retired and Senior Volunteer Program (currently known only as RSVP).

METHODOLOGY

The study methodology included several steps. We conducted a literature review to understand the demographic patterns projected for the future. After reviewing reports and publications, we spoke with people directly involved in the work of the Senior Corps programs and with others active in research or practice in the field of volunteering to determine current strengths and limitations of the programs and prospects for the future. Telephone interviews were conducted with national experts, directors of national voluntary organizations, project directors of Foster Grandparent Programs, Senior Companion Programs and RSVP, and with Corporation State Directors. We held several focus group discussions with project directors in the Southwest cluster, North Central cluster, and the Atlantic cluster of the United States during their 2001 conferences. In total, we interviewed or conducted focus group discussions with five experts in the field, three project directors or staff of national voluntary organizations, ten state directors of the corporation, and with twenty-six SCP, twenty-seven FGP, and forty-five RSVP project directors.

The following sections discuss the Senior Corps programs in the context of volunteering and then describe the programs. Drawing on information from nearly 100 interviews and focus groups, we then discuss the strengths of these programs, how changes in the elderly population might affect them, and factors limiting the programs as well as prospects for the future.

DESCRIBING NATIONAL SENIOR SERVICE: THE SENIOR CORPS VOLUNTEER PROGRAMS

Volunteer programs under the Corporation for National and Community Service can provide a structured framework for attracting older volunteers with diverse backgrounds, including those with strong interpersonal skills as well as others with rich professional backgrounds. The three volunteer programs FGP, SCP, and RSVP offer different types of volunteer opportunities for older volunteers. FGP provides support to children, mostly one-on-one. SCP provides one-on-one services to frail elderly so that they can live independently in the community. RSVP volunteers help frail elderly to continue to live independently, assist seniors in preparing income taxes, help young children learn to read, and meet other community needs.

According to Title II of the Domestic Volunteer Service Act of 1973 (Public Law 93-113), as amended and set forth in 42 U.S.C. section 5000, the purpose of the Senior Corps programs is to "empower older individuals to contribute to their communities through volunteer service, enhance the lives of the volunteers and those whom they serve, and provide communities with valuable services." In 1993 these programs became part of the Corporation for National and Community Service.

Altogether, the three Senior Corps programs involve more than a half million Americans over the age of fifty-five in service activities. One important question is whether these programs can meet the challenges of demographic changes in the U.S. population and evolving community needs in future years.

THE FOSTER GRANDPARENT PROGRAM

The Foster Grandparent Program (FGP), initiated in 1965, became part of the ACTION program under the Domestic Volunteer Service Act of 1973. About two-thirds of the financial support for the FGP is provided by the federal government. FGP projects also receive matching funds from other sources, including states, local governments, and private entities. FGP affords low-income volunteers ages sixty and older with opportunities to provide a range of supportive services to children and youths with special and exceptional needs. About 90 percent of FGP volunteers are women. Most foster grandparents serve as mentors, tutors, and caregivers in schools, day care centers, Head Start programs, and centers for mentally retarded/challenged individuals. Others work in hospitals, shelters for runaways and abused mothers, and other types of programs for children and youths. Participants are encouraged to serve in literacy and substance abuse programs, to mentor children, and to serve children of the incarcerated and children in foster care. FGP volunteers establish sustained, supportive relationships with children and youths to improve their physical, mental, and social development and facilitate independent living. These activities keep FGP volunteers physically and mentally active and improve their self-esteem, while making a valuable contribution to the community.

FGP grants are provided to public and private nonprofit organizations. A staff member of the sponsoring organization, acting as an FGP project director, administers the program and manages relations with the volunteer workstations to which the foster grandparents are assigned. FGP volunteers are trained and supervised by station supervisors at their workstations. In 2003, foster grandparents volunteered through 344 projects (Senior Corps, FGP National Overview, 2004a). In return for twenty hours of service per week, FGP volunteers receive small tax-free stipends, an annual physical examination, accident liability insurance, reimbursement for transportation expenses, and on-site meals during service. In 1999, 15 percent of the foster grandparents were reported to be between sixty and sixty-four years old, 49 percent were between sixty-five and seventy-four years, and 30 percent were between seventy-five and eighty-four years old. Five percent of the foster grandparents were over eighty-five years old. Foster grandparents in 2003 were somewhat older than in 1995. The ages of the clients served ranged from zero to five years (40 percent), six to twelve years (45 percent), thirteen to twenty years (13 percent), and more than twenty-one years (1 percent).

THE SENIOR COMPANION PROGRAM

The Senior Companion Program (SCP) is also means tested and pays a stipend to participants for their help in maintaining the independence of seniors. Senior companions provide companionship to older people who are often isolated, geographically or socially. Each senior companion helps to keep several seniors independent. Serving an average of twenty hours per week, companions provide assistance in paying bills, housekeeping, and arranging for transportation. They take clients on errands to the grocery store, the bank, and to medical appointments. They provide relief for caretakers, prepare light lunches, and perform simple housekeeping chores.

The age distribution of senior companions has not changed markedly over time. In 1999, 16 percent of the senior companions were between sixty and sixty-four years old, 51 percent were between sixty-five and seventy-four years, and 28 percent between seventy-five and eighty-four years. Five percent of the senior companions were eighty-five years or older. In 2003, 13 percent of the senior companions were between sixty and sixty-four years, 48 percent were between sixty-five and seventy-four years, and 34 percent between seventy-five and eighty-four years (Senior Corps, SCP overview, 2004c).

THE RSVP PROGRAM

RSVP is a national network of older Americans that provides volunteer service to communities through myriad local organizations. RSVP is the largest of three programs in the National Senior Service Corps. Anyone age fifty-five and over may serve as an RSVP volunteer. RSVP has neither income eligibility nor hours-of-service requirements, and provides no stipends for program participants.

The program addresses community-defined needs, operating through grants to local public and private nonprofit organizations (referred to as sponsors) in communities throughout the country. A member of the grantee organization serves as RSVP project director. Project sponsors provide funding (in addition to the federal grants) and are responsible for administrative and other in-kind support for project staff, for community fund-raising, and for community relations. Sponsors are expected to select and support a project advisory council. The broad categories of service areas are health and nutrition, education, community and economic development, human needs services, environment, and public safety. RSVP volunteers serve in community organizations (referred to as volunteer stations) such as hospitals, nursing homes, food banks, schools, and libraries.

In 1999, RSVP operated through 764 projects varying widely in size, type of sponsoring organization, number of stations, number of volunteers, and the population density of the areas served. Half of the budget for the program in 1999 came from nonfederal sources. The median RSVP grant was about $43,000. Approximately 75 percent of the RSVP volunteers were women, 4 percent were between ages fifty-five and fifty-nine years, 11 percent were between sixty and sixty-four years, 38 percent between sixty-five and seventy-four years, and 36 percent were between seventy-five and eighty-four. In 2003, RSVP volunteers served through 759 projects. The age ranges of the RSVP volunteers in 2003 were similar to those in 1999 (Senior Corps, 2004b).

STRENGTHS OF THE SENIOR CORPS PROGRAMS

The value of the three Senior Corps programs to communities and to volunteers themselves is well-documented. Senior Corps volunteers can and do provide a variety of services to the community that would otherwise be costly and difficult to find. Many project directors express frustration about their ability to modernize programs due to constraining regulations and tight budgets. They are trying, nevertheless, to improve the efficiency of project operations, use limited budgets more effectively, and maintain programs that are attractive to their volunteers and to members of the community. Projects under the stipended programs (FGP more so than SCP) are struggling to recruit volunteers in an economic environment where only 9 percent of older persons are income eligible to participate as volunteers in contrast to over 30 percent in the early days of the program. Project directors in both urban and rural areas are having difficulties in finding enough volunteers to meet the needs in their communities (Thomas & Silva, 2002; Bass, Caro, & Chen, 1993).

Not only are services of volunteers in all three programs in demand in communities across the country, but seniors themselves are said to benefit from participation. Several project directors mentioned that they have seen their volunteers blossom in their new "careers." Many develop speaking skills or acquire new knowledge of programs for seniors and other topics. Especially in rural areas, volunteers are able to escape from isolation and depression by becoming involved in useful activities.

Over time, the scope of the contributions made by Senior Corps volunteers has broadened in response to increasing requests for assistance. Senior Companions, working with frail elderly one-on-one, have increased their emphasis on keeping people out of institutions and in their own homes. Foster Grandparents, which originally focused on caring for handicapped children or children with developmental disabilities in institutions, have moved into other settings and activities. They now assist children with their homework, play games, help with hygiene and table manners, and are sometimes called upon to deal with behavioral problems. Foster grandparents today work in a greater variety of places where children are present. Some agencies are able to take children who would otherwise be institutionalized because they have foster grandparents to help. Moreover, grandparents provide continuity since their turnover rates are often lower than those of younger staff members.

Of the three Senior Corps programs, RSVP offers volunteers the most diversity and flexibility. The FGP and SCP programs play a more "hands-on" role in managing volunteers. RSVP might be described as a placement service, where potential volunteers can call one phone number for access to many different opportunities, instead of contacting organizations directly. Some RSVP volunteers prefer to apply their professional skills or previous work experience to their volunteer assignments, while others (some retired teachers for example), chose to do something entirely different with their time. Volunteers are involved in specific activities such as assisting people to complete federal income tax returns, providing information for seniors on long-term care insurance and other health topics, playing in bands, monitoring pollution levels in streams, and organizing and assisting with periodic events.

Although FGP and SCP project directors are concerned that requests for services are becoming too demanding for the typical level of skills possessed by their volunteers, many of whom are women with no previous work experience, RSVP is seeking even more complicated and interesting assignments for their recruits. Project directors report that RSVP volunteers want more challenging assignments than they are usually offered such as the opportunity to assist in administering non-profit organizations or grant writing, or the chance to use degrees in planning, engineering, and other technical subjects. In some instances, RSVP volunteers may be more apt than foster grandparents, for example, to have skills that enable them to assist with complicated homework assignments, tutor students in math or science, and handle children with increasingly more difficult behavioral problems. One project director noted that children who were considered as difficult twenty years ago are seen as normal now. If the demand for more skilled services continues, and RSVP responds, the organization might attract higher proportions of educated baby boomers, and ultimately redefine or displace the other two programs.

LIMITATIONS TO NATIONAL SENIOR CORPS GROWTH

For growth opportunities to materialize, the Senior Corps needs to make changes to overcome the problems faced by most projects in recruiting volunteers and running successful programs. Unless necessary changes are made, the Senior Corps programs may not continue to grow and might even experience a "natural death" while other organizations attract the baby boomer volunteers. Project directors have reported that already they seem to be losing volunteers to other programs which provide rewards that are more tangible and allow more flexibility. Project directors told us they were hampered by several specific limitations, most of which could be alleviated by larger budgets or fewer restrictions on the use of existing funds. One of them felt that the federal budget holds back growth.

Although project directors and state directors are eager to pursue new opportunities for growth, they are aware of many impediments to doing so. They believe that low budgets and restrictions on the use of funds limit project expansion and development and prevent them from adequately compensating volunteers for their services through stipends and expense reimbursements. The budget for Senior Corps programs has grown slowly over the past several years in relation to the rapidly increasing demand for volunteer services. In FY (fiscal year) 2002-2003, the federal budget for all three programs was $210,997,714, with $56,135,118 allocated for RSVP, $45,254,963 for SCP, and $109,607,633 for FGP (see Table 3.1). In 1999, the total budget was $170 million, split roughly in the same proportions. Across this same time period, the numbers of volunteers decreased by 3 percent in RSVP, and increased by 12 percent in SCP, and 13 percent in FGP (see Table 3.2).

TABLE 3.1. Budget allocations for the Senior Corps programs in 1999 and 2003.

	1999 budget in millions of dollars	2003 budget in millions of dollars	Proportion of budget in 1999	Proportion of budget in 2003
Foster Grandparents Program (FGP)	92	109	54%	52%
Senior Companion Program (SCP)	36	45	21%	21%
RSVP	42	56	25%	27%
Total	170	210	100%	100%

Source: Senior Corps, 2004a,b,c. Program overviews.

TABLE 3.2. Number of Senior Corps volunteers in 1999 and 2003.

	Number of volunteers in 1999	Number of volunteers in 2003	Increase in the number of volunteers from 1999 to 2003	Percentage change in the number of volunteers from 1999 to 2003
Foster Grandparents Program (FGP)	28,700	32,500	7,061	13
Senior Companion Program (SCP)	14,700	16,500	2,026	12
RSVP	485,000	468,600	−16,400	−03
Total	528,400	517,600	−7,313	

Source: Senior Corps, 2004a,b,c. Program overviews.

Some project directors resented the relatively large sums of money spent under the National Grants program for two other volunteer projects, claiming that the sponsoring organizations were given approximately $400 per volunteer, in contrast to $85 per volunteer for Senior Corps programs. Federal funds for the FGP and SCP are earmarked by Congress. Stipends for the volunteers make up 80 percent of the budget, with no flexibility to use some of the money for transportation or for other important functions even if money is left over when all volunteer service year (VSY) slots are not filled. There is much strategic maneuvering to fill VSY slots: sponsors guess how many extra volunteers to take on with the expectation that some will leave before the end of the year. Sometimes, however, the guesses are imprecise. Funds earmarked for volunteers or for other specific activities may have to be returned when they cannot be used as budgeted, even when needed for something else. There seems to be confusion among some project directors about the extent to which funds can be moved from one budgeted activity to another. A few directors stated that their district offices were able to transfer funds from one project to another that needed more money for the same function. Most directors, however, felt that the rules prevented them from using funds flexibly and thereby developing better programs.

Limited budgets and restrictive program rules impede projects. The effects of these constraints are explained in the following lists.

1. *Project directors are underpaid.* The salaries of project directors, determined by the sponsoring organizations' CEOs, were reported to be low compared with salaries offered for similar positions by other programs. The amount of work expected of project directors is not in keeping with their rates of pay; they must write proposals and raise funds, maintain relationships with other community organizations, and handle recruitment and training as well as manage projects. As a result, young people who join as project directors tend not to stay in the job for long. Low salaries not only encourage turnover but also decrease the pool of potential project directors.

2. *Projects have too few staff to recruit volunteers, engage in long-term planning, and keep up with paperwork.* All project directors complained that they did not have enough staff. Many of them had only one assistant, sometimes employed only part-

time because of limited funds. Virtually all of them would assign one full-time person to recruit volunteers if given the luxury of more help. Some project directors found that paperwork and reporting consumed an inordinate amount of time. If additional staff were available, many of these activities could be easily delegated. Because of the burdens of keeping up with day-to-day activities, some project directors said that they did not have time "even to think of expansion."

3. *Projects lack funds for staff travel.* All project directors reported that travel budgets were very limited. We were told that although regulations stipulate that volunteers should be supervised regularly, it is difficult to pay close attention to them if there is no money to pay for travel. Traveling to volunteer sites can be especially costly when a project covers a large territory. Projects must hold fewer training sessions when travel budgets are limited.

4. *Volunteer stipends are too low.* The tax-free stipend offered under the Senior Companion and Foster Grandparent programs, now at $2.65 an hour (taxfree), has not kept up with inflation. When the programs started in 1965, the stipend was closer to the minimum wage. Often volunteers who are eligible to be foster grandparents or senior companions because of their low incomes need more than the stipend to live on. As one project director said, "We're asking folks to do a lot, and we don't give them much." Project directors reported that they often inform seniors about available part-time jobs paying closer to $10 an hour at local stores because they cannot "in good conscience" ask them to donate time when they are so desperately poor. Most project directors would like to have the stipend increased by "a reasonable amount" and closer to the minimum wage. Many would prefer to keep the stipend just below the minimum wage to retain the voluntary character of the program and not turn it into a form of employment. One person did suggest raising the stipend to its original minimum-wage level.

5. *Funds for expense reimbursements are limited.* In addition to paying low stipends, some project directors reported that they did not have sufficient funds to reimburse volunteers for their expenses. In many rural areas, volunteers often drive thirty miles or more one way to reach a client and are not reimbursed

for travel. In programs that do pay travel expenses, some have recently increased allowances to 34.5 cents a mile whereas others reimburse only 25 cents. Under certain circumstances, volunteers can receive up to $2.00 toward the cost of a lunch, scarcely enough for even a simple meal anywhere in the country. Some projects provide payments for expenses only when they are requested, hoping that volunteers will not know that they are entitled to such reimbursements and will not ask. As another strategy to cut down on expense reimbursements, programs have introduced a cap ($100) on the amount a volunteer can claim in a month.

6. *Income eligibility guidelines are too low.* Volunteers in Foster Grandparents and Senior Companion programs must meet income standards to participate in the programs. Generally, participants must have very low incomes. Income eligibility criteria are updated annually. Project directors in these stipended programs, and especially in Foster Grandparents, believe that they will not be able to attract many of the new baby boomer retirees under the current income guidelines. Many reported that they constantly turn away able and willing people whose incomes are just above the current thresholds.

Why is there such difficulty in recruiting volunteers when there are still so many potential volunteers with very low incomes? Almost all of the longtime project directors have noticed a dramatic change in the types of volunteer candidates they encounter today in contrast to several years ago. Today, very low-income seniors are more likely than in the past to have disabilities, low levels of education in contrast to the society at large, or to have health problems that preclude a half-time volunteer commitment. If they are physically able, many potential low-income applicants need paid employment to make ends meet. Consequently, many elderly people who would meet the eligibility requirements simply cannot meet the demands of the programs, or cannot afford to. Many project directors claim that whereas they once had waiting lists of volunteers, they must now search continuously for new recruits.

The CNCS has been aware of the desire of project directors and others in the Senior Corps programs for more flexibility. In 1998, it launched a demonstration project titled Experience Corps for Independent Living (ECIL) that tested new ways of attracting qualified and experienced volunteers age fifty and over to volunteer. This program, similar to the Senior Companion program, relaxed many of the more stringent requirements of the program to significantly expand the size and scope of volunteer efforts for independent living services for frail elders (Rabiner, Koetse, Nemo, & Helfer, 2003). Volunteers did not have to serve twenty hours every week. Instead, they could serve up to twenty hours a week or even no hours during some weeks. Volunteers did not have to meet income-eligibility guidelines, and had a number of service options. By the second year of the demonstration, the projects had generally realized their goal of expanding the supply of independent living services to frail elders and their families, while providing opportunities for leadership, more flexible hours, and rewards to volunteers (Rabiner et al., 2003). This demonstration showed that changes in requirement could improve the capacity of the program to meet community needs and satisfy volunteers.

THE FUTURE OF NATIONAL SENIOR SERVICE

A number of possibilities for expanding the services and responsibilities in each of the three Senior Corps programs have been identified. In addition, there is a potential for broadening the base of volunteers by recruiting underrepresented categories of retirees. In 1994, men represented only 15 percent of senior companions and 11 percent of foster grandparents. Even if caregiving is not typically an area of strength, men have talents to offer children in sports activities, hobbies and recreation, and can be good companions to adults. Minorities are generally well-represented in the stipended programs (36 percent), although their recruitment is a continuing challenge. Compared with the two stipended programs, only 11 percent of RSVP volunteers, however, are drawn from minority groups. These two population groups, men and minorities, represent important potential sources of recruitment for the Senior Corps programs.

In addition to changes in Senior Corps programming, there are several conflicting social trends that may have an impact on the nature of senior service and the types of older volunteers over the next few decades. Research demonstrates that wealthier and healthier older people are more likely to volunteer. At the same time, they are likely to lead more active lives including traveling and visiting vacation homes, thereby leaving less time for volunteering. Seasonal migration is increasing, with larger numbers of elderly spending winters in warm climates and returning to cool places in the summer.

In 1999, only 39 percent of volunteers preferred to perform services at a scheduled time; all others preferred sporadic or irregular activities. Certain types of volunteer activities are more difficult to perform when continuity is broken, such as establishing relationships that people count on or taking on responsible positions in organizations. Yet healthier, wealthier, and more highly educated volunteers want activities that are not merely routine. Such activities often require commitment and some degree of regularity.

Some older people are easing into retirement while retaining part-time employment. Recently, the decreasing pool of younger job applicants has been a boon to older workers and, to the extent this need continues, part-time employment into the retirement years may flourish. This trend may have several implications. One study suggests that people committed to work find retirement without a steady amount of paid employment unsatisfying (Hooker & Ventis, 1984). Consequently, they may not be ready to take on unpaid responsibilities such as volunteering. On the other hand, as Bradley (2000) suggests, older people may volunteer so that they can acquire new skills. After they become accomplished in new areas, however, older people may then seek new, paid, full-time or part-time jobs rather than continuing to donate their services.

Volunteer organizations need to accommodate and attract new generations of volunteers as well as provide useful services to the community. Baby boomers who have been used to autonomy and independence may not be willing to fit into the existing volunteer positions available through the CNCS. It will be a challenge for the CNCS to examine its current programs and make changes to accommodate the baby boomers who will soon retire and to effectively utilize their services to meet the demands of society.

Current trends including increases in the socioeconomic status and in the health and longevity of the aging population, increasingly more diverse groups of minority elderly, changes in current volunteering patterns and motivations of volunteers all provide opportunities for the Senior Corps to revitalize its programs and recruit new participants. Programs will need to focus on areas of interest to volunteers, more appealing reward structures, and on other ways of shaping programs to benefit the new volunteer populations and the broader community.

REFERENCES

American Council of Life Insurance. (1999). *Long term care insurance: Choice you can afford.* Washington, DC: Author.

Bass, S.A., Caro, F.G., & Chen, Y.P. (1993). *Achieving a productive aging society.* Westport, CT: Aubern House.

Boraas, S. (2003). Volunteerism in the United States. *Monthly Labor Review,* 126(8): 3-11.

Bradley, D. B. (2000). A reason to rise each morning: The meaning of volunteering in the lives of older adults. *Generations,* 23(4): 45-50.

Caro, F.G. & Bass, S.A. (1995). Increasing volunteering among older people. In S.A. Bass (Ed.), *Older and active: How Americans over 55 are contributing to society.* New Haven, CT: Yale University Press.

Dye, D., Goodman, M., Roth, M., & Jensen, K. (1973). The older adult volunteer compared to the non-volunteer. *The Gerontologist,* 13: 215-218.

Ellis, S.J., & Noyes, K.H. (1990). *By the people.* San Francisco: Jossey-Bass.

Fischer, L.R., Mueller, D.P., Cooper, P.W., & Chase, R.A. (1989). Older volunteers: A discussion of the Minnesota Senior Study. *The Gerontologist,* 31: 183-194.

Fischer, L.R. & Schaffer, K.B. (1993). *Older volunteers: A guide to research and practice.* Newbury Park, CA: Sage Publications.

Height, D.I., Toya, J., Kamikawa, L., & Maldonado, D. (1981). Senior volunteering in minority communities. *Generations,* 5: 14-17, 46.

Herzog, A.R. & House, J.S. (1991). Productive activities and aging well. *Generations,* 15(1): 49-54.

Herzog, A.R., Kahn, R.L., Morgan, J.N., Jackson, J.S., & Antonucci, T.C. (1989). Age differences in productive activities. *Journal of Gerontology: Social Sciences,* 44: S129-S138.

Hooker, K. & Ventis, D. (1984). Work ethic, daily activities and retirement satisfaction. *Journal of Gerontology,* 39: 478-484.

Hunter, K. & Linn, M. (1981). Psychosocial differences between elderly volunteers and non-volunteers. *Aging and Human Development,* 12: 205-213.

Independent Sector. (1988). *Giving and volunteering in the United States.* Findings from a national survey conducted by the Gallup Organization. Washington, DC: Author.

Independent Sector. (1999). *Giving and volunteering in the United States.* Findings from a national survey conducted by the Gallup Organization. Washington, DC: Author.

Kilpatrick, J. & Danziger, S. (1996). *Better than money can buy: The new volunteers.* Winston-Salem, NC: Innersearch Publishing, Inc.

Kim, S.Y. & Hong, G.S. (1998). Volunteer participation and time commitment by older Americans. *Family & Consumer Sciences Research Journal,* 27(2): 146-166.

National Council on the Aging. (1981). *Older volunteers: A national survey.* Washington, DC: Author.

Ozawa, M.N. & Morrow-Howell, N. (1988). Services provided by elderly volunteers: An empirical study. *Journal of Gerontological Social Work,* 13(1): 65-80.

Rabiner, D.J., Koetse, E.C., Nemo, B., & Helfer, C.R. (2003). An overview and critique of the Experience Corps for Independent Living Initiative. *Journal of Aging & Social Policy,* 15(1): 55-78.

Scheibel, J. (1996, Winter). Recruiting the over-the-hill-gang for national service. *Social Policy,* 30-35.

Senior Corps. (2004a). Foster Grandparent program. National overview. Available online at http://www.seniorcorps.org/research/pdf/overview_fgp.pdf.

Senior Corps. (2004b). RSVP national overview. Available online at http://senior corps.org/research/pdf/overview_rsvp.pdf.

Senior Corps. (2004c). Senior Companion program. National overview. Available online at http://www.seniorcorps.org/research/pdf/overview_scp.pdf.

Thomas, C. & Silva, P. (2002). Senior Corps futures study. Final report.

Thompson, E. & Wilson, L. (2001). The potential of older volunteers in long-term care. *Generations,* 25(1): 58-63.

Chapter 4

Expanding Youth Service Concepts for Older Adults: AmeriCorps Results

Karen Harlow-Rosentraub
Laura B. Wilson
Jack Steele

INTRODUCTION

The decline in government or public-supported services due to budget deficits, unstable economies, and increased demands of defense/security spending has required the worldwide not-for-profit sector to fill the gaps in social service provision (Abraham, Arrington, & Wasserbauer, 1996; Bass & Caro, 2001). The not-for-profit sector currently represents the world's eighth largest economy—ahead of such countries as Russia, Spain, and Canada. It supports 19 million workers and relies on the input of more than 10 million volunteers (WorldVolunteerWeb, 2004). To meet current and increasing needs associated with rapidly changing demographic characteristics, the continuing recruitment and long-term involvement of a large volunteer workforce are critical international policy concerns.

Policy entrepreneurs from many countries have studied various volunteer efforts headed by governments or nongovernmental organizations (NGOs) to determine successful models for capturing the capacities represented by an increasingly aging and experienced population. The traditional volunteer of the past was a homemaker with available time for structured and scheduled volunteer work. Experts predict that twenty-first-century volunteers will search for short-term assignments with high levels of personal rewards (Grantmakers Forum, 2003). Their activities may be associated with continuing employment and the need for flexible hours for participation.

Concern has been voiced in America that the baby boomer generation (born between 1946 and 1964) has failed to volunteer at the levels of its parent generation. The lower level of volunteer participation is partially explained by the larger number of women in the workforce with fewer hours to devote to the traditional model of volunteering. Yet individuals in this birth cohort represent a rich source of potential contribution because of their increased life expectancy after retirement, higher educational levels, and improvements in health status over older cohorts (Magee, 2004). Recent studies by the Bureau of Labor Statistics have identified volunteer rates at 28.8 percent of the U.S. population who have worked within an organization in the past twelve months (Urban Institute, 2004). Other researchers have expanded the definition of volunteering to include services provided within families or communities but not associated with service to a specific organization. Participation rates increase an additional 36 percent among the age fifty-plus cohort (AARP, 2004) when this expanded definition is applied. Both AARP (2004) and Hart (2002) have found support for the idea that incentives would double the rate of volunteering among the baby boomers.

Programs offering incentive-based motivation for volunteering include the Peace Corps and AmeriCorps/Vista among others. A movement toward service learning as a crucial component of the volunteer experience and community capacity building have also provided impetus and models for consideration in building a larger volunteer corps to provide needed services in the future. Participating in a national service program could be especially attractive to older adults. Service was an expectation and was integrated into their neighbor-helping-neighbor mentality as modeled through their parents' generation. This concept has, to some extent, been lost or diluted with urban sprawl, increased mobility, and migration patterns. However, the only readily available intervention to meet the ever-increasing social and health needs of our nation is the cohort of older adults. It is the largest single and fastest growing age cohort. Vastly untapped, this generation has the potential to reduce the service gaps in our country through sustained volunteer service. They have the most amount of leisure time of any age group, have disengaged totally or partially from paid work, and are seeking meaningful ways to use their time to add value to their life.

The University of Maryland's Center on Aging has spent the past fifteen years developing evidence-based strategies for building a vital and responsive volunteer workforce from the enormous resource base of the baby boomer generation. As early as 1992, the University of Maryland Center on Aging and its National Eldercare Institute on Employment and Volunteerism formed a working group with AARP, the Administration on Aging, the American Red Cross, the National Council on the Aging, and the Points of Light Foundation to assess the future of senior volunteerism.

The development of this capacity-building project focused on life-long learning, meaningful volunteer roles, and the provision of purposeful social networking as the means to attract a well-educated population of volunteers, most of whom voiced no interest in association with any program labeled "senior" or "older American." The name for the project, Legacy Corps, was selected purposefully and was the result of the input of many different planning and focus groups. The linkage of some formal educational training with the provision of a service that requires the use of skills that go far beyond the traditional "envelope stuffing" perceived by many to be the role of volunteers was the mechanism to draw in more volunteers who might be willing to provide more intensive service (ten to twenty hours a week) over a longer period of time than the average volunteer. The intent was to find meaningful ways to engage the fifty-plus population in responding to unmet community needs.

One critical service shortage expected in the coming years involves the provision of respite care to family caregivers who attempt to meet the needs of vulnerable family members by keeping them in their own homes or supporting them in their communities. In the 1980s and early 1990s, studies found that more than 80 percent of all caregiving occurred outside the purview of the formal sector, and was provided by spouses, children, grandchildren, other relatives, friends, or neighbors. More recent analyses indicate that this has dropped to approximately 70 percent. Further changes in this pattern of informal caregiving would result in a potentially crushing demand for formal, in-home services in a network already overstretched to meet the needs of an increasingly large demographic cohort. Yet families report feeling stretched to the limit by caregiving responsibilities. In response to this growing national crisis of unmet home-health care needs, and in particular in-home respite care for older adults, the

University of Maryland Center on Aging developed a service model for older adults to serve in their local communities through the AmeriCorps Program.

The AmeriCorps Program, created in 1993, is one of several federally funded national service programs administered through the Corporation for National and Community Service. The primary objective of AmeriCorps is to support people and organizations using citizen service as a strategy to meet critical national and community needs and to foster an ethic of civic responsibility (Corporation for National & Community Service, 2004). AmeriCorps purposely uses the word *member* rather than *volunteer* to signify participation in a national network of programs under a common set of goals and objectives. In 2004 approximately 75,000 members served in over 900 programs nationwide.

The basic tenets of AmeriCorps are best described by four common goals:

1. *Getting things done* through direct and demonstrable service that helps solve community problems in the areas of education, public safety, environment, and other human needs;
2. *Strengthening communities* by bringing together Americans of all ages and backgrounds in the common effort to improve our communities;
3. *Encouraging responsibility* by enabling members to explore and exercise their responsibilities toward their communities, their families, and themselves; and
4. *Expanding opportunity* by enhancing members' educational opportunities, job experience, and life skills. (Corporation for National & Community Service, 2002)

AmeriCorps has traditionally been viewed as a career pathway for younger citizens (ages seventeen to twenty-five) aspiring to go to college or as a way to reduce their existing school loans. In this context, members agree to engage in community service projects such as environmental, educational, public safety, or other human needs for a set number hours (1,700 or less) in a twelve-month period. Members receive a modest living allowance that is usually paid monthly. In addition, in exchange for their service, members are eligible to receive an educational award through the National Service Trust Office. The combined service commitment coupled with an educational incentive has been highly successful in attracting younger citizens and instilling in them a greater sense of civic responsibility.

The University of Maryland Center on Aging set out to design and test a service model targeting older adults (aged fifty and older) to see if they too would commit to providing sustained service in their communities within the framework of the AmeriCorps program. Several questions needed to be asked.

- What changes would need to take place to attract older adults to sustained community service?
- Would they in fact commit to engaging in service for at least fifteen to twenty hours a week?
- How would this program impact their connection and commitment to their community?
- Would there be any changes in cognitive development or health status?

To answer these and other questions, a series of evaluation instruments were developed to measure these yet unknown outcomes.

Through a national, competitive process in 2001, the University of Maryland Center on Aging was awarded a grant by the Corporation for National and Community Service as an AmeriCorps National Direct Service Organization. A National Direct Service Organization must provide service in at least two states. This award would now provide the framework to begin to answer many of these questions. In the first year, a pilot study of three sites in two states was completed. The second year included eight sites. Findings from these eight sites comprise the findings reported later in this chapter. These programs have now expanded to eleven sites in seven states.

A goal of the comparison study design was to select diverse organizations and populations to determine both the flexibility and adaptability of the service model for older adults. Program participants range from those receiving Medicaid to those of moderate income representing diverse ethnicities (e.g., African American, white, Hispanic, Russian immigrants). The organizations under which programs operate include faith-based, not-for-profit, public, and governmental entities. All applicants to the program (primarily fifty-plus adults) must complete a competitive application and screening process. Members are then asked to sign a contract to complete at least 450 hours of in-home respite service in one year. An outcome-based, life-long learning educational curriculum, limited to 20 percent of service hours, is a core component of the program. The new generation of baby boomers is attracted to continuous learning opportunities, which, when coupled with meaningful service, result in increased life satisfaction.

Members are provided a monthly living allowance to offset some of the costs related to service assignment. Members may also use this stipend to pay for housing costs, food, medicines, or transportation. Ongoing reflection sessions integrated into the training component allow for meaningful social connections, provide a forum for collective problem solving, and stimulate greater community service among the members. At the end of their initial preservice training, members and their families participate in a formal graduation ceremony that recognizes their achievement and transitions them into their direct service assignment.

Upon completion of their 450 hours of service, members are eligible to receive an educational award. This award allows them to further pursue their individualized, lifelong learning plan, which may lead to full- or part-time employment opportunities. All of these program elements combined provide added value and life satisfaction for older adults and increase the likelihood that they will provide intensive and sustained community service thereby expanding community capacity to meet unmet human service needs.

From its inception, the Legacy Corps for Health and Independent Living Model has been committed to tracking measurable outcomes for the program that look at organizational and community changes as well as changes that occur within the volunteer or the service recipient. McBride, Pritzker, Daftary, & Tang (2004) have criticized youth volunteer programs as failing to adequately track this full measure of outcomes and focusing more on the volunteer. The research design for Legacy Corps was selected to demonstrate the capacity of the fifty-plus population within a national service structure, AmeriCorps, which initially focused on seventeen- to twenty-five-year-olds. It was intended to provide evidence of the potential value of further expansion of AmeriCorps with volunteers over age fifty.

This chapter describes the first full year of data collection (Year Two) in eight sites for the Legacy Corps Model. The design of the project follows a quasiexperimental, nonequivalent-comparison-group panel design in the eight funded sites. Preliminary data were collected in year one from the three start-up sites, and a pilot evaluation report was submitted in December 2002. This chapter focuses on the second year of activities and expands that analysis to eight sites, describing selected achievements to date.

The purpose of the evaluation is to track outcomes for three different groups, each on a different time line. The design allows for organizational outcomes tracking over a three-year period to determine changes in waiting lists for needed respite services, recruitment of additional nonstipended volunteers, and, for the final year, a third organizational outcome is an increase in the number of collaborative partnerships in the community to address the needs of dependent elders. Management changes made to accommodate volunteers are also recorded. Cumulative change over time will be reported in the final evaluation report (Harlow, Steele, & Wilson, 2005).

The second group for which outcomes are tracked is the members. The database for year two contains responses for 275 members with an additional fifty available from the first-year pilot study. Measures of relationship to community, political involvement, physical and emotional health and life satisfaction, types of volunteer activities and likelihood of continuation, as well as cognitive change involving learning new information are tracked for these individuals.

The third group studied for changes in outcomes is caregivers and care recipients. In respite care, the primary consumer of service is the caregiver. Extensive sets of measures of stress and burden and intentions to continue providing care have been collected both from the adult caregiver and whenever possible from the care recipient. A one-year follow-up study of caregivers has been completed and a second follow-up was completed in summer of 2005.

The remainder of this chapter summarizes the findings from the baseline and first follow-up study at eight participating sites.

SITE COMPOSITION OF LEGACY CORPS ACTIVITIES

The eight sites that are the focus of this chapter represent publicly funded agencies such as area agencies on aging (Salt Lake City AAA), faith-based organizations (Lutheran Social Services of Illinois, Lutheran Social Services of Minnesota, and Alpert Jewish Family and Social Services in Miami), and nonprofit organizations, Mather Life-Ways (Chicago), Miami Latino Elderly, West Palm Beach AAA, and Tampa AAA (see Tables 4.1 and 4.2).

The sites are fairly equal in size with the largest concentration in Lutheran Social Services in Illinois and West Palm Beach and the smallest in Mather and Salt Lake City AAA. The organizations coordinating the sites are predominantly not-for-profit (54.4 percent) with 35.54 percent faith-based and 10.5 percent public.

Who Are the Members?

At baseline, the largest concentration of members, 48 percent, was seventy-plus years of age. The age cohorts range from thirty-nine to eighty-nine with the Miami site focusing on a somewhat younger member group. Similar concentrations are identified for follow-up indicating successful tracking of members (see Table 4.3).

TABLE 4.1. Site composition for Legacy Corps activities.

Site	Percent
Luth. Soc. Serv. IL	18.9
West Palm	17.7
Tampa	14.2
Miami	13.0
AJSFCS Miami	12.7
Luth. Soc. Serv. MN	10.6
Chicago Mather	9.9
Salt Lake	9.9

TABLE 4.2. Agency types sponsoring Legacy Corps activities.

Type of agency	Percent
Nonprofit	54.4
Faith-based	35.4
Public	10.1

Almost two-thirds of the members were white, and just under one-fifth were Hispanic. More than 13 percent were African American (see Table 4.4).

Almost 15 percent of the members had completed a college degree, and an additional 14 percent had a master's, doctorate, or professional degree. Eleven percent did not complete high school or complete a GED certificate.

More than two-fifths were married with another 46 percent evenly divided between divorced and widowed status.

Almost 80 percent of the members were female.

Why Did the Members Join Legacy Corps?

Understanding an individual's motive(s) for volunteering is key to developing a program that achieves the goals of its volunteers, thus increasing the possibility that they will continue to participate and volunteer their time in the community or organization. Members identify multiple reasons for joining Legacy Corps. Desire to be involved in the community was named most often, followed closely by desire to help people or solve problems. However, when asked to identify the single most important reason for joining, members iden-

TABLE 4.3. Age composition of respondents.

Age in years	Baseline respondents	Follow-up respondents
Below 40	17.3	6.3
41-54	17.9	16.0
55-69	4.7	45.1
70 or over	29.8	22.5

TABLE 4.4. Racial composition of respondents.

Race	Baseline respondents	Follow-up respondents
African American	13.3	12.2
Hispanic	17.7	18.2
White	65.9	66.5
Other	3.1	2.9

tified helping people or solving problems in the community substantially more often than any other response (43.6 percent) (see Tables 4.5 and 4.6).

What Is the Relationship to the Home Community?

The goals of Legacy Corps are to impact the volunteer, the service recipient, the agency, and the community. The relationship of the volunteers to the community and the level of their participation reflect

TABLE 4.5. Reasons for joining Legacy Corps.

Reasons	Percent
To be involved in community	77.6
To help people or solve problems in community	77.3
To utilize my knowledge and skills	66.8
To join a network of others committed to community service	62.1
To expand knowledge and skills	56.3
To explore future job or volunteer service opportunities	42.2
To work with people who have different backgrounds than I have	35.7
To eventually move into paid employment	18.1
Other	9.7

TABLE 4.6. Most important reason for joining Legacy Corps.

Reasons	Percent	Rank
To help people or solve problems in community	43.7	1
To be involved in community	15.3	2
To join a network of others committed to community service	12.3	3
To utilize my knowledge and skills	10.4	4
To expand knowledge and skills	6.3	5
To explore future job or volunteer service opportunities	5.6	6
Other	3.4	7
To eventually move into paid employment	2.2	8
To work with people who have different backgrounds than I have	0.7	9

civic engagement and the potential to keep influencing the community after involvement in stipended activities is ended. A critical part of the evaluation is to measure civic engagement and political participation over time to determine the relevance of the Legacy Corps experience and to determine its potential for building more long-term commitment and capacity.

A scale devised from five questions measured relationship to community at baseline and again at follow-up observation about six months into the project. Figure 4.1 identifies the five individual questions and the changes on each individual measure. On each measure the follow-up responses show fewer unsure, disagree, or strongly disagree ratings. This shift indicates a change toward stronger community attachment for each single measure within the scale.

On the cumulative scale, scores on relationship to the community improved a statistically significant five standard deviations from baseline to first follow-up using paired-sample T-tests. Mean score at baseline was 18.8 and at follow-up was 20.6 (see Figure 4.2).

All age groups show substantial improvement over time in relationship to their community.

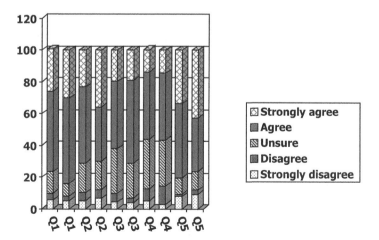

FIGURE 4.1. Relationship to community. Q1 = I feel that I (make/made) a contribution to the community; Q2 = I (have/had) a strong attachment to my community; Q3 = I (have/had) a good understanding of the needs and problems facing the community in which I serve; Q4 = I (am/was) aware of what can be done to meet the important needs in my community; Q5 = I (feel/felt) I have the ability to make a difference in my community.

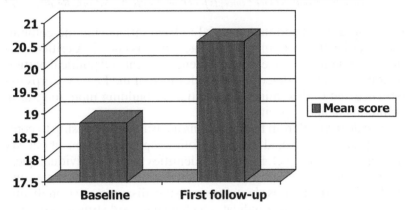

FIGURE 4.2. Changes in community relations scale.

Almost all racial/ethnic groups improve over time with Hispanic respondents showing the greatest gains. Respondents in the "other" category reported a slightly lower mean at baseline (–.1 change) but the small numbers in that racial category suggest the need for more respondents before making policy interpretations.

With the exception of Lutheran Social Services of Minnesota, all sites registered substantial gains. However, the Minnesota measure is believed to be nonrepresentative due to a printing error in the questionnaire which made responding to those five questions more difficult for those members and thus is eliminated from this comparison.

Gains were noted for all agency types with public organizations registering the largest changes.

POLITICAL ACTIVITY AND CITIZEN INVOLVEMENT AMONG MEMBERS

Civic engagement also involves political activity and involvement in community groups. A scale consisting of fourteen widely used measures of citizen/political involvement was included in the baseline with additional questions focusing on expected levels of involvement after leaving Legacy Corps. These probes focus on voting participation at national, state, and local levels as well as involvement in a variety of community-based organizations, advocacy groups, community projects, rallies, and protests.

Political activity and involvement vary significantly by most of the demographic characteristics of sample respondents. Males report significantly higher scale scores than females (34.8 and 32, respectively). Divorced respondents report a high of 36.3 versus singles at 26.5. The association with education is significant and linear with better-educated respondents substantially more involved than individuals who had less than high school or a high school equivalency education. The youngest respondents report a substantially lower scale score, 16.6, compared with the fifty-five- to sixty-nine-year-old group at 35.7 (see Table 4.7) Hispanics are significantly less involved than other racial/ethnic categories (19.0) compared to a high for white respondents at 36 (see Table 4.8). Strongly associated, significantly different scores at the different sites range from a low of 16.5 at Miami Latino Elderly to a high of 37.8 at West Palm Beach AAA (see Table 4.9). Faith-based organizations report higher levels of involvement than other agency types.

A scale that measured expectations for future political and civic involvement was used in the baseline since the timing for the first follow-up (five to six months) would probably preclude respondents'

TABLE 4.7. Involvement in political activities prior to Legacy Corps by age.

Age in years	Mean score
Below 40	16.6
41-54	29.9
55-69	35.7
70 or over	34.1

TABLE 4.8. Involvement in political activities prior to Legacy Corps by race.

Race	Mean score
African American	34.4
Hispanic	19.0
White	36.9
Other	34.3

TABLE 4.9. Involvement in political activities prior to Legacy Corps by site.

Site	Mean score
Luth. Soc. Serv. IL	37.2
West Palm	37.8
Tampa	35.0
Miami	16.5
AJSFCS Miami	34.9
Luth. Soc. Serv. MN	35.1
Chicago Mather	35.5
Salt Lake	32.4

ability to make many behavioral changes in participation outside the realm of the required 450 hours associated with Legacy Corps. The questions comprising the scale asked about the likelihood that respondents would participate in a number of activities that were similar in nature to the activities described on the political involvement scale. Although expectations of involvement in full-time work or part-time work were asked, they were not included in the scale. As such, the scale does not measure actual change, but rather the respondents' expectations that they might be involved in these kinds of activities after finishing their responsibility to Legacy Corps.

The future involvement scale showed lower levels of expectations among the youngest cohort with the highest among the fifty-five to sixty-nine years cohort, but the differences were not significant. The scale also does not vary by gender, marital status, or agency type. Significant changes are noted for education, race, and site. Individuals with two years of college or less report the highest expectations for participation followed by those who have completed graduate or professional education and those who have a high school equivalency certificate or less than high school education (Table 4.10). Highest levels of expectation are noted at Lutheran Social Services of Illinois and Lutheran Social Services of Minnesota (Tables 4.10 and 4.11). Highest expectations among racial groups are noted for African Americans with whites reporting the lowest mean score (Table 4.12).

TABLE 4.10. Expected level of future involvement by educational category.

Educational category	Mean score
Less than high school or equivalent	29.7
High school graduate	26.1
Less than 2+ years college	30.7
2+ years college or vocational	27.6
College graduate	27.4
Graduate/professional	30.4

TABLE 4.11. Expected level of future involvement by site.

Site	Mean score
Luth. Soc. Serv. IL	32.2
West Palm	28.3
Tampa	28.2
Miami	29.3
AJSFCS Miami	26.0
Luth. Soc. Serv. MN	30.3
Chicago Mather	27.3
Salt Lake	29.0

TABLE 4.12. Expected level of future involvement by race/ethnic group.

Race	Mean score
African American	32.6
Hispanic	29.0
White	29.0
Other	31.0

What Is the History of Members' Previous Volunteer Activities?

An important aspect of developing increased community capacity is identifying new participants as members and volunteers. Programs that draw from already committed volunteers may change the nature of service provision but do not necessarily represent increased capacity for the nonprofit sector. The Legacy Corps project does attract individuals who have volunteered their time previously to other organizations, but it also represents a strong component of "new" skills and capacities. In addition, prior to Legacy Corps, the vast majority had volunteered from zero to five hours per week or less often. The Legacy Corps commitment averages twelve-plus hours a week, indicating that it is possible to attract volunteers to serve more hours.

More than one-fifth of the members had never volunteered, and two-fifths had been involved an average of one to five hours per week or less often. Eleven percent of the members had been involved for twenty hours or more per week prior to joining Legacy Corps.

Caregiving also represents a type of volunteer activity within the family or friendship structure. More than one-fourth had no experience with caregiving, but almost one-third (30.5 percent) had previously spent twenty or more hours per week in this activity prior to joining Legacy Corps.

How Do the Volunteer Activities Affect the Health of Members?

Literature on volunteering has long touted the positive effects of involvement on health. Some recent studies, however, have questioned whether there is a point at which the positive "return" decreases or stops and involvement can become too demanding or potentially damaging (Morrow-Howell, Hinterlong, Rozario, & Tang, 2003). This point has been argued in Musick, Herzog, & House (1999) who found that volunteering has a positive effect on mortality for those that volunteer forty hours a year or less. Van Willingen (2000) work suggests that a positive effect may disappear after 100 hours per year. These studies highlight an important point because policy initiatives such as AmeriCorps and the Boomer Corps (Magee, 2004) require substantially more hours per year than some suggest.

The health results tracked in this study all focus on individuals who volunteered under AmeriCorps requirements (450 hours per year). Measures taken from the Health Quality of Life (HQOL) module on the Behavioral Risk Factor Surveillance System were utilized to determine changes in physical and mental health status (see Table 4.13). At follow-up, the following were noted:

- Almost 70 percent of the members reported the same or more days when they felt good or energetic (24 percent improved). The change from baseline to follow-up was statistically significant.
- Almost three-quarters of the members reported the same number or fewer days when their health was not good. This positive outcome was also statistically significant.
- Almost 90 percent remained stable or improved on the measure of number of days they could not perform their normal activities or duties.
- On self-reported health status, 80 percent remained stable or improved and 20 percent declined. The improvement from baseline to follow-up was statistically significant.
- More than four-fifths remained stable or improved on the measure of number of days they felt sad or depressed.
- Three-quarters remained stable or improved on the measure of number of days they felt worried or tense.
- Sixty-three percent remained stable or improved on numbers of days they were unable to sleep or rest.
- Eighty-five percent reported stable or improved self-assessment of emotional or mental health. This change was statistically significant.

TABLE 4.13. Change in health quality of life measures.

Health quality of life	Stable	Improve	Decline
Days felt good, energetic	45.1	23.6	31.3
Days physical health not good	61.4	12.4	26.2
Days could not perform normal duties	79.3	9.0	11.7
Changes in self-reported health status	68.0	12.2	19.7

What Kind of Cognitive Change Can Be Demonstrated for Members?

The goals of Legacy Corps include the improvement of service provision as well as the improvement of quality of life for the volunteers/members. The acquisition of new knowledge addresses both the service sector and member changes. Producing volunteers who improve in their knowledge skills can provide better, more well-informed services. Furthermore, increasing volunteers' knowledge serves as a cognitive exercise that directly affects their mental functioning and quality of life.

Knowledge about aging and related service issues increased a statistically significant 7.24 points from baseline to first follow-up observation. These changes are measured by objective test questions developed from the training and include covering the process of providing direct service as well as content questions focusing on necessary understanding of the aging service recipient (see Figure 4.3).

Members were also asked to evaluate their self-reported assessment of knowledge about aging issues at baseline and again when the knowledge instrument was administered at follow-up. Members described their understanding as increasing an average of 2.2 points on a 10-point scale. This change was also statistically significant (see Figure 4.4).

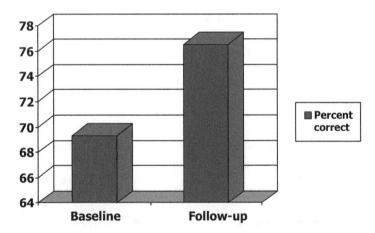

FIGURE 4.3. Change in knowledge score from baseline to follow-up observation.

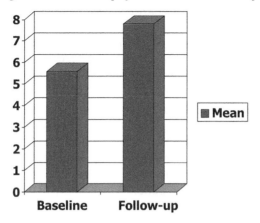

FIGURE 4.4. Perceptions of knowledge about aging issues.

CONCLUSIONS

Although the changes presented here reflect less than six months in the field for most members, significant changes can already be documented. The learning/training process that is an integral part of the Legacy Corps model combined with strategic placement in a direct service activity that benefits both elders and caregivers creates an increasing level of attachment and sense of community involvement in members. The changes in scale scores from baseline to follow-up are substantial and significant.

The recruitment process in each site identified individuals who vary widely in political and civic interests and involvement at the beginning of the project. Differences are noted on almost every demographic variable. The greater interest and involvement in political and civic activities for the older participants presents an important opportunity for mentoring and role modeling. The disengagement from the political process for younger Hispanics shows a potential, major focus that future training might address. A particularly encouraging finding is the high level of expectations for future involvement noted for African-American members.

Health status measures for the members also show encouraging trends of improvement. Both self-reported physical and emotional health measures identify significant change over time. In addition, specific health status measures such as days not feeling physically well or days feeling full of energy showed change in a positive and healthy direction. This finding is particularly important in view of some research that suggests the beneficial health outcomes associated with volunteering may be linked to much lower levels of involvement (i.e., 100 hours per year) rather than the 450 required by the Legacy Corps/AmeriCorps model.

Members demonstrated increased knowledge about aging issues and methods of caring for dependent elders. The objective measure of cognitive change/improvement is supported by members' perceptions that they are mastering new material. Further refinement of analyses as the project progresses will introduce age categories such as the "dotcom" generation, generation X, baby boomers, young old, and mature old. Recruitment at Legacy Corps sites is focusing on building multigenerational teams, thus providing more participants who fit into the younger categories. Their motivation and expectations for participation can help better shape the policies that will attract future volunteers.

The concept of political activity will be redefined into two separate measures—political involvement and civic involvement. Individuals who participate in one type or the other can be compared to those who are "dual activists." Studies of motivation will link volunteers' reasons for joining a Legacy Corps project with longer-term participation and satisfaction with their experiences. New incentive structures will be offered in addition to the living allowance and educational benefit, which will enable comparisons of the success of various reward structures.

The addition of these independent and dependent variables into a mix of comparison groups expanded to new sites and types of participants will strengthen the already rich base for policy research. The Legacy Corps projects offer a unique opportunity to help build evidence-based recommendations to guide the development of blueprints for successful civic engagement and lifelong learning opportunities for baby boomers as well as other age groups.

REFERENCES

AARP. (2004). Time and money: An in-depth look at the 45+ volunteers and donors. Available online at http://www.aarp.org.

Abraham, I., Arrington, D., & Wasserbauer, L. (1996). Using elderly volunteers to care for the elderly: Opportunities for nursing. *Nursing Economics,* 14: 232-238.

Bass, S. & Caro, F. (2001). Productive aging: A conceptual framework. In N. Morrow-Howell, J. Hinterlong, & M. Sherraden (Eds.), *Productive aging: Concepts and challenges.* Baltimore: Johns Hopkins Press.

Corporation for National & Community Service. (2002). *AmeriCorps program director's handbook.* Washington, DC: Author.

Corporation for National & Community Service. (2004). *2005 AmeriCorps guidelines.* Washington, DC: Author.

Grantmakers Forum. (2003). The costs of a volunteer: What it takes to provide a quality volunteer experience. Available online at http://www.GFCNS.org.

Harlow, K., Steele, J., & Wilson, L. (2005). *Civic engagement, lifelong learning and baby boomers: A three-year evaluation.* College Park, MD: University of Maryland Center on Aging.

Hart, P. (2002). *The new face of retirement: An ongoing survey of American attitudes on aging.* Washington, DC: Civic Ventures.

Magee, M. (2004). *Boomer corps: Activating seniors for national service.* Washington, DC: Progressive Policy Institute.

McBride, A., Pritzker, S., Daftary, D., & Tang, V. (2004). *Youth services: A global perspective.* Working Paper No 04-12. Global Service Institute Center for Social Development. St. Louis: Washington University.

Morrow-Howell, N., Hinterlong, J., Rozario, P., & Tang, F. (2003). Effects of volunteering on the well-being of older adults. *Journal of Gerontology: Social Sciences,* 58B(3): 5137-5145.

Musick, M., Herzog, A., & House, J. (1999). Volunteering and mortality among older adults: Findings from a national sample. *Journals of Gerontology Series B: Psychological Sciences and Social Sciences,* 54(3): S173-S180.

Urban Institute. (2004). Volunteer management capacity in America's charities and congregations: A briefing report. Washington, DC: Author.

Van Willigen, M. (2000). Differential benefits of volunteering across the life course. *Journal of Gerontology: Social Sciences,* 55B: 308-318.

WorldVolunteerWeb. (2004). 29 million workers can't be wrong. Available online at http://www.worldvolunteerweb.org.

PART III:
LIFELONG LEARNING
AND CIVIC ENGAGEMENT

Chapter 5

Civic Engagement
and Lifelong Learning Institutes:
Current Status and Future Directions

Sharon P. Simson
Laura B. Wilson
Karen Harlow-Rosentraub

INTRODUCTION

Lifelong learning has emerged as a central focus of the active life-style of the baby boomer generation. Well-educated, healthy, having discretionary income, and accustomed to meaningful work and community involvement, this generation looks to the future as a time that offers new opportunities to continue learning and civic engagement (Federal Intra-Agency Forum, 2000; Nordstrom, 2004; Wilson, Steele, D'heron, & Thompson, 2002; Thompson & Wilson, 2000). The lifelong learning movement has been spearheaded by Elderhostel and its Elderhostel Institute Network (EIN), an association of over 300 Lifelong Learning Institutes (LLIs) in the United States. LLIs have provided hundreds of thousands of active adult learners age fifty-plus with the opportunity to enrich their lives through educational activities such as study groups, classes, courses, lectures, and field trips. LLIs enable participants to pursue year-round learning in their home communities through programs affiliated with their local colleges and universities.

Although these educational activities have been the core focus of LLIs, engagement in community-based volunteer service has been emerging as a complementary pursuit. Elderhostel has expanded its educational offerings to include opportunities for service learning in the United States and abroad. An opportunity exists for LLIs to expand their mission in home settings and to enhance the social capital of their communities through a combination of lifelong learning with civic engagement. Although conferences, articles, reports, and EIN communications have heightened our understanding of the educational mission of LLIs, formal assessment has not occurred previously concerning the expansion of the functions of LLIs into community-based volunteer service.

This chapter discusses findings about the current lifelong learning activities and involvement of LLIs in community-based volunteer service leadership. It presents the views of LLI leaders regarding future initiatives that could combine lifelong learning with community-based volunteer service leadership. The chapter explores the implications of LLIs expanding their organizational mission to include engagement in the civic affairs of their communities and increasing in social capital. An agenda is presented for future LLI development and research on combining lifelong learning and civic engagement.

THE EDUCATIONAL MISSION
OF LIFELONG LEARNING INSTITUTES

The first Lifelong Learning Institute, the Institute for Retired Professionals, was founded in 1962 by a group of retired public school teachers at the New School for Social Research in New York City. Additional institutes that replicated or adapted the New School model were established at college and university campuses throughout the country during the 1960s, 1970s, and 1980s. Building on this momentum, the Elderhostel Institute Network (EIN), a voluntary association, was created by Elderhostel in 1988 to extend the learning-in-retirement concept to additional people and campuses and to strengthen and support the effectiveness of established institutes. The number of Lifelong Learning Institutes associated with EIN has grown dramatically from 32 affiliates in 1989, 101 affiliates in 1992, 175 affiliates in 1995, to over 300 affiliates in 2005. Approximately 60,000 people are members of the various LLIs affiliated with EIN (Elderhostel Institute Network, 1995, 2004).

According to EIN, two basic premises define a Lifelong Learning Institute: ownership (learners develop their own college-level, educational programs) and community (organizational structure distinguishes the institute as an educational community of older learners).

Peer learning, collaborative leadership, and active participation by members are fundamental. Institutes typically share a set of common goals and characteristics. They offer college-level course work, usually on a noncredit basis; operate as member-led organizations with an identity and purpose created by members who choose to join; promote open membership and participation without regard to previous levels of formal education; and create cocurricular learning programs that combine courses with social events, membership meetings, and field trips (Elderhostel Institute Network, 1996).

A curriculum based on a study-group approach to lifelong learning is the core of the LLI experience. Study groups are similar to college courses and offer opportunities for serious study and learning. They differ from regular college courses in that they do not award grades, require tests, offer academic credit hours, or lead to degrees. They are chosen, designed, and led by peer educators who are LLI members, university faculty and staff, and community members who are knowledgeable in the subjects they lead. They are conducted through a variety of formats: seminars, discussions, presentations, lectures, and field trips. In keeping with models of effective adult learning, study groups emphasize experiential learning and encourage active participation rather than passive listening. Participants help to shape the content and learning style of a study group according to their interests and learning objectives. Preparation at home is common.

Study groups can cover a wide variety of subjects such as literature, languages, the arts, history, science, mathematics, social sciences, business and economics, computer technology, and other topics of interest to members. Usually, the LLI calendar corresponds with the semester schedule of the affiliated university or college. Study groups meet for two to three hours each week for up to fifteen weeks during the two semesters of the academic year. The size of the group may vary from a small seminar of five to a lecture for a hundred. In addition to the core study groups, LLIs may offer cultural activities, social events, university privileges, university alumni memberships, and educational field trips and travel. Many LLIs draw on the programs and resources offered by their affiliated colleges and universities and local communities. Membership fees may range from a few dollars for an event to several hundred dollars for a year's all-inclusive membership. LLI membership may range from about 50 members to 500 members or more.

THE CIVIC ENGAGEMENT MISSION OF LIFELONG LEARNING INSTITUTES

Lifelong Learning Institutes are established and developed by volunteers and are member run. Even the LLIs that receive staff and facility support from colleges or universities rely heavily on volunteer leadership. The goals, policies, activities, and operations of LLIs are determined and implemented by members. Hundreds and often thousands of hours of volunteer service are needed each year to maintain an LLI and to enable it to grow and thrive. Some LLIs are exploring opportunities to contribute as organizations to their local communities. They are considering the responsibilities of their LLIs to their communities and ways that they could be engaged in external community-based volunteer service which would enhance social capital in their communities.

Civic engagement can be defined as "being a concerned citizen, involved in helping others in the community" and "involvement in community activities" (Putnam, 2000, p. 25). Putnam states that "social capital refers to connections among individuals—social networks and the norms and reciprocity and trustworthiness that arise from them" (Putnam, 2000, p. 19). Social capital is defined further by the Saguaro Seminar on Civic Engagement in America (2001a) as follows: "Social capital refers to the value of the social networks embodied in various communities (both geographically and communities of interest), and the trust and reciprocity that flows from those networks." The Seminar cites eleven facets of social capital: social trust, interracial trust, conventional political participation, protest politics participation, civic leadership, associational involvement, giving and volunteering, faith-based engagement, informal socializing, diversity of friendships, and equality of civic engagement at a community level. *Better Together,* a publication of the Saguaro Seminar (2001b), maintains

> the national stockpile of social capital has been seriously depleted over the past 30 years. By virtually every measure, today's Americans are more disconnected from one another and from the institutions of civic life than at any time since statistics have been kept. Whether as family members, neighbors, friends, or citizens, we are tuning out rather than turning out. This decline was found to affect Black, White, Native, Latino, and

Asian Americans; males and females; young and middle-aged; city dwellers, suburbanites and rural residents; professionals and blue collar employees. (p. 5)

In marked contrast to this overall decline in civic engagement, Putnam (2000) has found that the cohort population which continues to be engaged is older adults. People age fifty and older have sophisticated knowledge and skills and a high level of civic commitment that can enhance the social capital of their local communities (Thompson & Wilson, 2000). Institutions such as the University of Maryland and its Center on Aging have pioneered models that combine lifelong learning and civic engagement for the fifty-plus age group. Its research has found that programs can combine lifelong learning and civic engagement and that each activity complements and enriches another activity. The University of Maryland Center on Aging has established leadership institutes that train people age fifty-plus not only to acquire specific skills but also to develop a broad perspective about community affairs and their roles as leaders. They apply their lifelong learning to community-based service leadership that impacts their communities and influences social policy (Wilson and Simson, 2003; Wilson et al., 2002). This chapter reports the results of research that explores lifelong learning and civic engagement activities of Lifelong Learning Institutes.

METHODS

Subjects

The 303 Lifelong Learning Institutes that were invited to participate in this study are affiliates of the Elderhostel Institute Network. Directors of these institutes were selected as respondents because of their organizational positions, experiences, historical perspectives, and leadership roles. Previous research of the investigators indicated that LLI directors were appropriate and reliable sources of information and insights about their LLIs (Simson, Thompson, & Wilson, 2001; Wilson & Simson, 2003). The researchers also discussed ideas about lifelong learning and civic engagement with the project manager of the Elderhostel Institute Network, Nancy Merz Norstrom.

She provided valuable insights about the organizational history and characteristics of LLIs and a list of potential research respondents.

Measures and Procedures

A letter describing the purpose and contributions of the research and a questionnaire were mailed to directors of all 303 Lifelong Learning Institutes. In addition, Nancy Merz Norstrom encouraged participation by sending several messages through the EIN e-mail discussion group *Forum*. These messages promoted the study and encouraged LLIs to complete the questionnaire. Follow-up phone calls, e-mails, and letters encouraged nonrespondents to participate.

LLI Respondents

A total of 109 leaders of the 303 LLIs responded. They represent a variety of membership sizes and years since being established. Five responses were submitted too late to be included. Directors of thirty-five LLIs (12 percent of all LLIs) indicated they were not responding because they viewed their LLIs as inappropriate respondents due to the nature of LLI lifelong learning activities (typically nonpeer-led lecture series, sporadic offerings, or travel ventures), small membership size, development stage, and/or their lack of experience as directors. Nearly 60 percent of the LLIs responding were established between 1969 and 1995.

The major growth in LLIs occurred in the past fourteen years (see Table 5.1). Size of membership varies (see Table 5.2).

Instrument

The questionnaire consisted of three parts: Part one presented seven questions about LLI organizational characteristics and current engagement in community-based, volunteer service leadership. Part two posed ten questions about potential future LLI engagement in community-based volunteer service leadership. Part three had two questions that asked respondents to think creatively about the impact and process of LLI engagement in community-based volunteer service leadership. A total of nineteen questions were asked: fourteen were forced choices, three were rating scales, and two were open-ended.

TABLE 5.1. Establishment of LLIs.

Year	Percent of LLIs
1969-1989	22.5
1990-1995	36.8
1996-1999	23.6
2000-2005	17.0

TABLE 5.2. Size of membership of LLIs.

Number of members	Percent of LLIs
1-199	34.6
200-499	35.5
500-999	23.4
1,000+	6.5

Data Analysis

Data entry and data analysis were performed using the Statistical Package for the Social Sciences (SPSS12). Descriptive statistics profiled the individual responses and multiple response formats were used to group the question series together as single, constructed variables in order to compare them by selected independent variables.

RESULTS ABOUT CURRENT STATUS OF LLIs AND CIVIC ENGAGEMENT

To establish a context for the study of civic engagement and LLIs, directors were asked about the extent of their connections with their partner universities/colleges. LLIs are usually established on or near a university campus but physical location may or may not translate into a strong relationship with the university. Since universities often have a high level of commitment to surrounding communities, the extent of LLI connection is important. Over 70 percent rated the extent of the connections of their LLIs with their university as very high or high. Only 7.5 percent rate the extent of connection as low or very low. When these responses are translated into a mean score with a possible range of 1 to 5, the average for all respondents is 3.89, indicating a tendency toward viewing connections with universities and colleges in a positive light. In addition to understanding the extent of the connection of LLIs to universities, it is also relevant to understand how this connection is viewed regarding its impact on the success of the LLIs. The findings indicate that the importance of university/college connections to the success of an LLI is perceived very positively with a mean score of 4.26 out of a possible five. Over 85 percent rated this connection as very important or important. Although the size of the LLI does not significantly impact the responses, the age of the program does. The oldest programs (established between 1962 and 1995) rank the importance of the connection higher than those established between 1996 and 1999. The relationship to age is not linear, however, since those LLIs established since 2000 report higher ratings of importance, more closely approaching those ratings of older LLIs (see Figure 5.1).

The most common types of connections LLIs have with universities/colleges are use of university facilities such as libraries and dining halls and use of meeting space. A majority of respondents reported that members attend programs at university/college partners and that the institutions provide faculty staff and lead study groups. Approximately 30 to 40 percent reported that faculty/staff serve on LLI advisory committees or boards, LLI members volunteer services

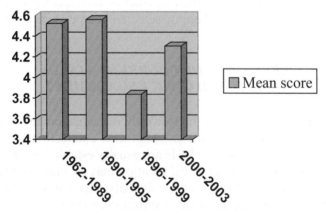

FIGURE 5.1. Mean ratings of importance of connection to universities/colleges.

TABLE 5.3. Nature of connections between LLIs and partner universities/colleges.

Type of connection to university/college	Percent
University/college provides meeting space	82.6
Use university facilities (i.e., dining hall, library)	82.6
Attend programs at university/college	67.9
Faculty/staff lead LLI study groups	53.2
University/college provides staff	53.2
Faculty/staff serve on LLI advisory committee/board	41.3
Attend courses offered by the university/college	38.5
Volunteer services to university/college	38.5
Faculty/staff are LLI members	33.9
Engage in intergenerational activities with students	29.5
Participate in university/college research projects	19.3
Hold membership in alumni association	14.7
Participate in service learning	9.2
Not connected with university	1.8

to university/college departments and programs, faculty/staff are LLI members, and LLIs engage in intergenerational activities with students (see Table 5.3).

In terms of engagement in their communities, 31.2 percent of respondents reported that their LLIs are engaged in community-based, volunteer service as part of LLI missions or functions compared with 61.5 percent negative responses and 7.3 percent that are planning such opportunities for the future. Respondents commented on reasons for their LLIs not being engaged in the community.

> It seems most of our members join our LLI for educational purposes and have their volunteer activities related to other organizations.

> We find that our members come to our program for courses. They already volunteer extensively in others parts of their lives such as church, neighborhoods, family, etc. Community-based volunteer service, in general, is not part of our mission.

> There are numerous well-organized, well-staffed volunteer groups in our city of which our students are a part. We are a new organization

and still at work on building a strong and stable program providing opportunities for lifelong learning customized to our needs (fifty-plus semi and retired). Many of our members volunteer countless hours to the community through other venues such as churches and other organizations that may be a better place for that.

The larger LLIs and the older LLIs reported more involvement in community-based volunteer service as part of their mission than the smaller and newer LLIs. Over 40 percent of the respondents for LLIs with memberships of over 500 stated that community-based volunteer service is part of their mission. In contrast, only 18.9 percent of respondents from LLIs with 1 to 199 members and 31.6 percent of respondents from LLIs with 200 to 499 reported community-based volunteer service as part of their mission. Nearly 42 percent of the respondents for the oldest LLIs, established in 1962-1989, stated that community-based volunteer service is a part of their mission. In contrast, 28.2 percent of respondents from LLIs established in 1990-1995, 28 percent established in 1996-1999, and a low 16.7 percent established in 2000 and later report community-based volunteer service is part of their mission.

Engagement in community-based volunteer service is implemented by LLIs through a variety of activities. Approximately one quarter of the respondents stated that their LLIs post opportunities for community-based volunteer service for members, partner with community-based organizations to offer volunteer service opportunities, and partner with universities/colleges to offer volunteer service opportunities. Only about 9 percent reported combining service learning activities with volunteer service in community-based organizations or conducting their own volunteer programs that serve the community (see Table 5.4). One respondent made this comment about engagement in the community: "We have an extensive volunteer program, RSVP, that sends our members in many different directions if they wish to do community service."

RESULTS REGARDING THE FUTURE
OF LLIs AND CIVIC ENGAGEMENT

When thinking about the future of LLIs, directors were asked to rate the importance of engagement by their LLIs in community-based volunteer service. Less than 20 percent of the organizations described

TABLE 5.4. Current engagement in community-based volunteer services.

Activity	Percent
Post opportunities for community-based volunteers	26.6
Partner with community-based organization to volunteer	24.0
Partner with university/college	21.1
Recruit volunteers for community-based volunteer service	18.3
Inform about web opportunities for volunteer services	11.9
Combine LLI with volunteer service in community-based organization	9.2
Conduct own volunteer services for community	8.3

involvement in community-based volunteer service as important to their future. A quarter were undecided, however. The potential interest, then, is slightly less than half of the total who already view involvement positively or are neutral about the issue. No significant variance was noted by size or age of organization. The younger organizations did report higher levels of interest but not at a statistically significant rate.

Among the seventy-seven agencies who did identify reasons they might become engaged in community-based volunteer services, the grouped variable that described all responses together identified more than two-thirds who linked volunteering with enhancing diversity of programs. More than half indicated they might become involved as a result of member interest, and almost half indicated they might become involved to enhance educational activities and experiences. Low on the list for reasons for future civic engagement of LLIs are research opportunities and financial incentives (both at 9.1 percent) (see Table 5.5).

Respondents from seventy-eight organizations identified one or more ways that they might learn about opportunities for community-based volunteer civic engagement. Among those organizations, a large majority identified their own members as major resources (79.5 percent). Others identified contacts initiated by community-based organizations about opportunities (69 percent), networking (63 percent), newsletters (63 percent) and formal announcements from universities/colleges (see Table 5.6).

TABLE 5.5. Reasons for future engagement in community-based volunteering.

Why might LLI become engaged in community-based volunteer service in the future?	Percent
Would enhance diversity	64.9
Member interest	53.2
Community-based volunteer service enhances educational experiences	49.4
Education leads to community-based volunteer service	44.2
Invited by community-based organization	40.3
Interest in networking	32.5
Community-based volunteer service is part of mission	28.6
University might encourage community-based volunteer service	27.3
Adding new initiatives	27.3
Geographic accessibility	23.4
Program commitment to combine LLI learning with community-based volunteer services	22.1
Research opportunities	9.1
Financial incentives	9.1

TABLE 5.6. Learning about opportunities.

How might LLIs learn about opportunities for community-based volunteer services?	Percent
Community-based organizations contact LLIs about opportunities	69.2
Suggestions by members	79.5
Newsletters and annual reports	62.8
Announcements from universities	63.0
Networking	62.8
Newspapers, magazines	47.4
Participation on boards	46.2
Conferences and meetings	34.6
Directories with information about opportunities	29.5
Senior Corps Web-based information	14.1
Other Web-based resources	12.8

When asked, "With what organizations might your LLI become engaged in volunteer service in the future?" seventy-five LLIs suggested one or more organizations: art, music, drama programs, and elementary, middle, and high schools most often (58.9 percent); senior groups (56 percent); universities and colleges (48 percent); retirement organizations (47 percent); and libraries and literary groups (44 percent each) (see Table 5.7).

Sixty-nine organizations proposed specific ways they might become involved in the future. Sixty-one percent of those respondents

TABLE 5.7. Potential organizational linkages.

With what organizations might LLIs engage in the future for community-based service opportunities?	Percent
Art, music, drama organizations	58.9
Civic associations	34.2
Colleges or universities	47.9
Elementary, middle, or high schools	58.9
Environmental programs	30.1
Faith-based organizations	19.2
Fire rescue organizations	6.8
Government or political organizations	13.7
Health organizations	37.0
Homeland security	9.6
Human service agencies	23.3
Law enforcement agencies	8.2
Libraries	43.8
Literary programs	43.8
Military and veteran groups	16.4
National service programs	12.0
Nutrition programs	12.0
Professional associations	16.0
Retirement organizations	46.7
Senior groups	56.0
Unions	12.0
Youth groups	18.7

proposed partnering with a university/college to offer volunteer service opportunities, and almost three-fifths proposed posting opportunities for community-based volunteer service for members. Almost half would combine service learning activities with volunteer service in community-based organizations and would recruit volunteers for community-based service organizations. The major factor discouraging their LLIs from becoming engaged in community-based volunteer service is the fact that this type of volunteer service is not viewed as part of an LLI's mission. Other factors discouraging engagement cited by approximately 25 percent of respondents were "LLI members might not have the resources to be engaged," and "LLI members might discourage engagement."

Directors report a wide variety of services that LLI members might perform in community-based organizations with which their LLIs might become engaged. Activities mentioned include teaching, tutoring, and mentoring, cited by 47.7 percent of respondents, followed by board membership (37.6 percent). Services selected by 20 to 30 percent of directors include: hospitality, program activities, friendly visitor, communication, marketing, community relations, outreach, computer technology, counseling, and service learning. Respondents predicted engagement in community-based volunteer service will have four major impacts on LLI educational activities: attracting new members to enroll in educational activities (51.4 percent), increasing educational program visibility in community (50.5 percent), developing new educational activities (46.8 percent), and providing new leaders for educational activities (38.5 percent). Only 11 percent of directors concluded that engagement would have no impact. Over 45 percent of directors indicated their LLIs might consider designing activities (study groups, courses, lectures) to prepare members for engagement in community-based volunteer service.

An open-ended question asked directors to predict the impact that LLI engagement in community-based volunteer service might have on recruitment of baby boomers to participate in their LLIs. Respondents indicated that they are anticipating positive changes in their LLIs due to an influx of baby boomers. Among the responses about impact on recruitment were: change views of baby boomers about retirement that allows them to pursue learning that they can apply to active involvement in the community, greater number of members offering a wider diversity of topics that can be presented to a growing number of participants, learning acquired by doing and not just listening in a classroom environment, larger enrollment, high potential for growth, more balanced selection of activities to do in retirement, contact with a broader age range, and more interest by LLIs in providing opportunities for volunteer service.

Another open-ended question asked directors, "Thinking as creatively as possible, please tell us your ideas about the best ways to engage LLIs in community based volunteer service in the future." Respondents presented a wide variety of ways to move their organizations into engagement in their communities including the following:

> Bring leadership of the LLI on board. Sell members on the benefits of volunteering in the community through an LLI. Encourage local organizations to work actively with LLI. Have a volunteer fair with events, information, giveaways, etc.

> Service learning is a great undergraduate program with which we could form a partnership. I think some intergenerational programs may work well.

> Organize a mini-mall recruitment rally at which all groups needing volunteers would "sell" their project/mission/ideas.

> List opportunities on LLI Web page and newsletters.

> Provide meaningful opportunities to use their skills and talents.

> Interact with community groups through our speaker's bureau.

> Participate in advocacy groups that provide hope of community change and broader awareness, particularly of senior issues.

> Research opportunities for community service, share findings with the LLI membership, select several community organizations through a consensus polling, and connect with the chosen organizations.

> Partner with organizations that will use an LLI volunteer's time wisely. Engage in activities that are truly worthwhile and not just busy work.

DISCUSSION

The findings of this study demonstrate the current status of LLIs regarding both the planning for and practice of volunteer service associated with lifelong learning. The findings clearly indicate that

LLIs continue to have a very strong link to the college or university and view this link as important to their continued success as a lifelong learning unit. Note that the relationship between colleges/universities and LLIs is largely based on what might be termed a reciprocal, volunteer relationship. In addition to providing meeting space, the university shares faculty and staff for several different functions. The LLIs, in return, provide member volunteer services to departments, programs, and students ranging from administrative support and mentoring to participation as subjects in research experiments.

This degree of involvement and reciprocity is an important key to the future potential of LLIs in playing a key role as an entry point into meaningful and extended civic engagement for the fifty-plus population. College and universities have increasingly emphasized their service role in their own communities. This commitment has resulted in more active engagement by both faculty and staff. Of particular significance has been the growth of service learning as an accepted and visible component of the curriculum. According to Jacoby (1996),

> service learning is a form of experiential education in which students engage in activities that address human and community needs together with structured opportunities intentionally designed to promote student learning and development. Reflection and reciprocity are key concepts of service learning. (p. 5)

Since 1996 there has been a dramatic increase in the number of students, institutions, and communities engaged in service learning (Jacoby, 2003). LLIs are a relatively new part of campus life. They can model their practices on that of their host university. A natural part of continued growth for LLIs would be to follow the college trend and enhance their involvement with and service to the community.

The findings show that this trend toward greater community involvement does extend from the university into the LLI and could potentially continue to grow. The larger and longest operating of the LLIs are most involved in community service. Establishing a strong involvement with the community that complements the academic missions has been an iterative process occurring over time for colleges and universities. The clear academic mission is established first, followed by applications in the community including field experiences, service learning, and community service. A similar pattern may be evolving for LLIs.

This evolution toward service in LLIs is not, however, oriented toward the creation of new service or service learning opportunities. Instead, they appear to use existing organizations and opportunities and find ways to offer these options to their members. Although this approach represents a critical avenue toward helping lifelong learning members find service opportunities, it does not reflect the more demanding expectations that define baby boomers. Baby boomers entering volunteer service through LLIs will most likely be looking for a more expansive and multifaceted experience in civic engagement. LLIs have the capacity, especially in cooperation with their host institutions, to offer such opportunities and add a critical dimension to the community service landscape.

Do LLIs share this vision for the future? Overall, a small percentage of directors of LLIs report that civic engagement is important to the future of their organization. In keeping with the theme of the evolution of service and service learning, it is interesting to note that LLIs in existence for the longest time and those that are newest are most likely to see civic engagement as important to their future, although the differences are not statistically significant. The long-standing LLIs, as noted previously, have had more time to stabilize their academic component and like their host institutions, can now turn toward related activities. The newer LLIs are most likely to be ready for innovation and are being developed in an environment where civic engagement already has been defined and structured, thereby making it more likely to be a part of the LLI mission from the beginning rather than as a component of change. These newer programs may already see the necessity and value of program diversification in attracting a broader audience, particularly the baby boomers. Since more than three-fifths of the respondents view civic engagement as a means of offering greater program diversity, newer programs may have arrived at this conclusion by benefiting from assessment of existing programs before becoming established themselves.

The actions that LLIs might take regarding future involvement in civic engagement are responses to community demand. Volunteer organizations are seeking ways to fill their volunteer needs and are turning to LLIs to access their membership. Although LLIs have the potential to provide more creative and appropriate options to their membership, this outcome will not be realized until both staff and membership view lifelong learning and service as inextricably linked and shift the LLI mission accordingly. If such a shift takes place, corresponding service opportunities may emerge that go beyond the more traditional options that directors mention as potential areas for service for their LLIs. As LLI membership becomes more infused with baby boomers, LLIs may find it necessary to adapt programs and make use of the specialized skills and capabilities of this cohort. A natural shift may occur with creative activities designed by the members themselves. Many directors responding to this study could see civic engagement as a viable avenue for the future and were aware of how volunteer activity might serve both their membership and the community in valuable ways. To make this transition, specific pathways must be created that help LLIs initiate a shift in their mission to specifically increase opportunities for civic engagement. Some recommendations about how to create those pathways to combine lifelong learning with civic engagement follow.

FUTURE DIRECTIONS

Lifelong Learning Institutes have the opportunity to increase the social capital of their communities through civic engagement. The findings of this study suggest that this future must be shaped and defined now in order for LLIs to be prepared for such an expanded mission.

I. *National conference on Lifelong Learning and Civic Engagement.* The goal of this conference would be to train LLI leaders to design, develop, and implement programs for their LLIs that combine lifelong learning with civic engagement. Attendees would be exposed to the importance of civic engagement to the future success of their LLIs and to their connections with universities/colleges and their communities. The conference could be conducted under the aegis of the university service learning specialists and those specializing in civic engagement of the over-fifty population in partnership with the Elderhostel Institute Network. Topics could include the following:

A. What are civic engagement and social capital and what are their importance to today's society?
B. What do we know from research on lifelong learning and civic engagement?
C. What can we learn and apply from existing service learning program models of various age groups to LLIs?
D. What are LLIs already doing to combine lifelong learning and civic engagement? How will introducing these concepts help LLIs create a sustainable future?
E. How can LLIs develop partnerships that promote lifelong learning and civic engagement? Topics could include:
    1. Recruiting leaders and participants
    2. Identifying LLI mission and interests and community needs
    3. Selecting an appropriate goal for a partnership
    4. Designing a project to accomplish this goal
    5. Planning the project tasks
    6. Implementing the project
    7. Evaluating outcomes
    8. Planning long-term partnerships

A postconference, computer-based, communication network on this topic could be established so that LLI leaders could confer about their initiatives and provide mutual assistance. Conference sponsors could develop applied research instruments to follow the progress of LLI initiatives and report outcomes to LLIs. This conference could lead to increased engagement by people age fifty-plus in meaningful volunteer leadership positions throughout the country.

II. *Next Chapters life planning programs conducted by Lifelong Learning Institutes.* Following the *Next Chapters* model demonstration and program developed and implemented by the University of Maryland Center on Aging in 2002, Lifelong Learning Institutes could present *Next Chapters* programs that help people make a successful transition from work, family life, and community involvement into the "next chapters" of their lives (Wilson & Simson, 2002). Lifelong Learning Institutes could adapt the *Next Chapters* programs to meet local needs and enable people fifty-plus to utilize their time, talent, and expertise to engage in meaningful community affairs. *Next Chapters* is comprised of four programs that can be replicated by Lifelong Learning Institutes:

    A. *Next Chapters Seminars* focus on the most important topics and questions facing people age fifty-plus. These seminars can enable participants to review past chapters in their lives, review opportunities for lifelong learning and civic engagement, and formulate future plans.

    B. The *Next Chapters Retiree-to-Retiree Network* focuses on opportunities for lifelong learning and civic engagement through computer-based chat rooms that can be maintained by Lifelong Learning Institutes. These chat rooms enable retirees to share experiences, participate in discussions, solve problems, access informative lectures through distance learning, and receive newsletters on a special Web site.

    C. *Next Chapters Resource Directories* present organized information about opportunities for volunteerism, lifelong learning, and employment for people age fifty-plus who reside in specific geographical areas. Contributions for a directory can be solicited from business, government, military, universities and colleges, housing communities, health services, unions, cultural institutions, professional associations, and nonprofit service agencies. Data collection methods include mailed questionnaires, documents such as brochures and Web sites, telephone conversations, and e-mail and letter correspondence.

    D. *Next Chapters Opportunities Day* can be sponsored by Lifelong Learning Institutes. LLIs can invite retirement resource directory contributors to meet face-to-face with people age fifty-plus, present exhibits about their organizations, and recruit new participants for their activities. All of these programs in the *Next Chapters* model demonstration could be adapted by Lifelong Learning Institutes to address the needs and interests of their constituents.

III. *Lifelong Learning Institutes incorporated into active adult communities.* People age fifty and beyond are pursuing active lifestyles. They are interested in living arrangements that offer more than the usual recreational amenities and are seeking opportunities to pursue lifelong learning on site and to engage in meaningful volunteer service projects in the community. LLIs could partner with volunteer agencies to offer on-site programs in fifty-five-plus communities that promote service learning and active engagement oriented to meeting relevant needs in surrounding communities.

IV. *Intergenerational Residential College Lifelong Learning Institute.* Changing demographics, financial pressures, and community pressures are influencing colleges and universities to redefine their educational mission and target population to embrace the large baby boomer/mature adult population. The residential college model for undergraduates could be redesigned to address the needs and interests for intergenerational involvement of the baby boomers. This type of intergenerational residential college could bring new people, resources, and energy to campus. In addition to providing the usual apartments, common rooms, and amenities, the residential college could house an LLI and be the center for intergenerational lifelong learning and civic engagement programs for the campus and surrounding community. In keeping with the tradition and history of LLIs, the residential college LLI could be member run and offer peer-led study groups, cultural, and social events. Members could be eligible to use the libraries, performing arts and recreation centers, bookstores, and dining halls. Faculty and students could be invited to live in the residential college, participate in LLI study groups and programs, and conduct their own classes and activities on site. In addition, intergenerational engagement in college/university and community projects could be a core mission of the residential college. The baby boomer generation has considerable expertise and experience that could benefit the campus and community. The LLI could combine lifelong learning with the development of new skills and leadership training for volunteer community service. Projects could be intergenerational and involve faculty and staff. Partnerships could be formed with campus service learning programs and course credits could be awarded to students for participation. The residential college with its lifelong learning and civic engagement activities could increase social capital by bridging networks existing on

campus and in the community and contribute to an understanding and appreciation of the capacities of the fifty-plus
population.

V. *Partnership of Lifelong Learning Institutes with campus service-learning programs.* Many colleges and universities offer
service-learning programs to their students. Service learning
is defined as "experiential education in which students engage
in activities that address human and community needs together with structured opportunities intentionally designed to
promote student learning and development" (Jacoby, 1996,
p. 5). LLI members could join with campus service-learning
programs and offer their talent, time, and resources to enhance
the learning experience of students and increase service contributions to the community while benefiting from stimulating
contact with students. This partnership would increase social
capital by breaking down intergenerational stereotypes and
building trust, diversity of friendships, and informal contacts
between generations.

VI. *Summer, short-term Lifelong Learning Institute community-
based service projects.* Most LLIs operate according to the academic calendar of their affiliated colleges and universities.
LLIs typically do not schedule many activities during the
summer months. Although LLI members tend to be busy with
activities such as travel and family visits, they might be interested in a one- to two-week summer program that offers leadership and skill training which could then be applied to short-
term, meaningful volunteer service projects in their local
communities. Since the summer is also a time when children
are on vacation and need worthwhile activities, LLIs could
partner with schools, community agencies, and faith-based
organizations to develop and conduct productive intergenerational service programs for and with children. These community-based organizations could follow the study group model
and provide training that would expose LLI members to new
ideas and skills while preparing them for service projects or
prepare both generations to serve together in the community.
An LLI could expand this summer initiative to become an
Elderhostel program that would invite people from other
places to participate.

VII. *Partnership of a Lifelong Learning Institute with a community-based organization.* Although meaningful opportunities for service leadership exist in community-based organizations, specialized training and skills may be required to fill these roles. LLIs could identify such opportunities and invite organizations to provide the needed training through study groups at LLIs. LLI members could be connected with appropriate positions. Continuing training could be offered through future study groups. This type of arrangement could be a particularly useful way for community-based organizations to recruit LLI members to serve on their boards by offering training in areas such as fund-raising and management. Interorganizational relationships between LLIs and community-based organizations could lead to the evolution and expansion of goals and activities of all participating organizations.

VIII. *Lifelong learning, civic engagement and employment.* The baby boomer generation has many different expectations and plans for their "retirement" years. Many would like to keep both their minds and bodies active through continuing education and volunteer service. Some choose or must continue to work part-time in previous jobs or related positions. Others are interested in part-time or full-time paid employment in areas that require additional expertise and skills. Volunteer service and employment options may not be clear. Opportunities to acquire the necessary training may be unavailable.

One route to exploring employment options, developing skills, and acquiring experience is through training and meaningful volunteer service. LLIs could offer education that prepares the baby boomer generation for meaningful volunteer service positions along with a potential path to future paid employment. LLIs could expand their educational mission to partner with community-based organizations to conduct training programs and study groups that would impart marketable knowledge and skills to those seeking volunteer service and/or employment in the workplace. LLIs could arrange volunteer positions for trainees and provide supervision and continuing education. The expertise and experience gained from volunteer service could lead to paid employment that could benefit workers and community productivity.

Each of these proposed initiatives could be evaluated to determine their effectiveness and impact on target communities. Particular focus could be on how such programs work to attract baby boomers into LLIs and into appropriate service opportunities. Findings could be used to determine future initiatives that could increase social capital by combining lifelong learning with civic engagement. The future of LLIs may be significantly enhanced through these efforts to bring the community into the learning process and to bring lifelong learners into the community through specially designed opportunities which bring "life" into lifelong learning.

REFERENCES

Elderhostel Institute Network. (1995). Who we are. Durham, NH: Elderhostel Institute Network.

Elderhostel Institute Network. (1996, July). Institutes for learning in retirement: An overview of the ILR movement. Durham, NH: Elderhostel Institute Network.

Elderhostel Institute Network. (2004). Available online at http://www.elderhostel .org.

Federal Inter-Agency Forum on Aging-Related Statistics. (2000). *Older Americans 2000: Key indicators of well-being.* Washington, DC: Author.

Jacoby, B. (Ed.). (1996). *Service-learning in higher education: Concepts and practices.* San Francisco: Jossey-Bass.

Jacoby, B. (Ed.). (2003). *Building partnership for service-learning.* San Francisco: Jossey-Bass.

Nordstrom, N.M. (2004, August). EIN Monthly Newsletter. Available online at www.elderhostel.org.

Putnam, R. (2000). *Bowling alone.* New York: Simon & Schuster.

Saguaro Seminar on Civic Engagement in America. (2001a). *Benchmark survey.* Cambridge, MA: John F. Kennedy School of Government, Harvard University.

Saguaro Seminar on Civic Engagement in America. (2001b). *Better together.* Cambridge, MA: John F. Kennedy School of Government, Harvard University.

Simson, S., Thompson, E., & Wilson, L.B. (2001). Who is teaching lifelong learners? A study of peer educators in institutes for learning in retirement. *Gerontology and Geriatrics Education,* 22(1): 31-43.

Thompson, E. & Wilson, L.B. (2000). The potential of older volunteers in long-term care. *Generations,* 25(2): 58-63.

Wilson, L.B. & Simson, S. (2002). *Next Chapters retirement planning for the baby boomers.* College Park, MD: University of Maryland Center on Aging.

Wilson, L.B. & Simson, S. (2003). Combining lifelong learning with civic engagement: A university-based model. *Gerontology and Geriatrics Education,* 24(1): 47-61.

Wilson, L.B., Steele, J., D'heron, C., & Thompson, E. (2002). The leadership institute for active aging: A volunteer recruitment and retention model. *Journal of Volunteer Administration,* 20(2): 28-36.

Chapter 6

Legacy Leadership Institutes: Combining Lifelong Learning with Civic Engagement

Laura B. Wilson
Jack Steele
Sharon P. Simson
Karen Harlow-Rosentraub

BACKGROUND AND DESCRIPTION

Much of the current thinking about the aging of America focuses on how the country will pay for a growing population of elderly. Terms such as "gray peril," "greedy geezers," and "the hippopotamus in the living room" are perjorative labels that detract from the recognition of the potential resources that a growing cadre of better-educated and healthier retirees represent for the nation. Society's beliefs and public policies must continue to evolve away from traditional stereotypes, negative labels, and distorted perceptions about what it means to grow older. We must rethink and revise our assumptions about older adults. This challenge means we must create positive and meaningful service roles, raise the level of assumed expectations, and develop innovative service models that transfer lifelong skills acquired from the workforce to meaningful, community-based, volunteer civic engagement opportunities.

The futuristic demographic implications of an increasingly aging population will impact the sociological, psychological, health, and economic infrastructure of our society. From a demographic perspective, the numbers provide a wake-up call to action. In the United States, there are 34 million people or nearly 13 percent who are sixty-five-plus. This number will rise to 40 million by the year 2011. It is at this point that the first wave of 77 million baby boomers begin to turn sixty-five. By the year 2030, one in every five Americans (20 percent) will be over the age of sixty-five. An individual who is sixty-five years old today can expect to live for another eighteen-plus years. At the peak of the baby boomer generation, our national profile will reflect that of the state of Florida, where 18 percent of the current population is over the age of sixty-five (Treas, 1995). The implications of this impending wave of older adults with increased longevity requires society to respond with organized and innovative structures that will actively engage baby boomers and future aging cohorts in meaningful pursuits that are responsive to societal need.

The question that confronts us as organizations and individuals is how prepared are we to recognize these changes in the fabric of society? In what ways will nonprofit organizations, the traditional bastion for the volunteer service sector, need to change to attract a new generation of volunteers? How will baby boomers respond to these changes? What new resources are needed? What are the policy implications? What will happen if we continue to do what we have always done or do not make system changes which will encourage those nearing retirement to make a sustained volunteer commitment?

The advent of the baby boomer generation propels us to rethink and reframe our message about what "older" means. The baby boomer generation is unlike any other previous generation. They defy previous stereotypes about aging while seeking new, meaningful lifestyles. They are active individuals who have amassed considerable expertise, experience, and skills while making valuable contributions to all sectors of society, business, and industry, government and the military, education, family, and community (Treas, 1995). Collectively, theirs is a voice that has and will continue to affect public policy and consumer spending. They will redefine the meaning of retirement and leisure.

Shaped by a variety of shared experiences (e.g., Vietnam War, Watergate, Civil Rights movement, women's movement, and environmental movement), baby boomers reflect distinct life values that directly impact their expectations about the future. They are eternal optimists about the future exuding a "we can do anything" spirit, are individualistic in their personal pursuits, openly question authority, are reformers, are self-confident, and seek experiences that provide personal growth, meaning, and adventure (Keefe, 2001).

Baby boomers are better educated than previous generations. In 1995, only 14 percent of individuals between the ages of sixty-five and seventy-four were college graduates. In contrast, by the year 2025, an estimated 33 percent of this age group will be college graduates. Thirty-seven percent of baby boomers report that continuing their education is an important part of their retirement plan (Hart, 2000). What are the implications of this better-educated, future older generation? What role can universities and other institutions of higher learning play as baby boomers look to them to provide meaningful educational experiences? The baby boomer generation will seek out opportunities that engage them in continuous education for increased skills and knowledge. University-based educational opportunities that combine lifelong learning with meaningful civic engagement open new doors for exploration and have the potential to change policy based on national research.

How do these trends and issues impact our view of retirement? Retirement, by definition, is undergoing a social and cultural metamorphosis. The notion of retirement as it is traditionally practiced—a onetime event that permanently divides work from leisure—no longer makes sense (Dychtwald, Erickson, & Morrison, 2004). Retirement is much more than that. Boomer retirees want to make a contribution, try new things, be challenged, learn, and be productive. This new concept of retirement is now achieved through a combination of paid work, volunteer service, and personal pursuits (Dychtwald et al., 2004). This trend means that volunteer organizations and programs which perpetuate traditional low-functioning/low-skill roles, focus on organizational loyalty versus personal development, and expect long-term commitments from menial work will neither attract nor retain the better-educated, self-actualized, baby boomer retiree.

In addition to changing perceptions about what retirement means, society is also faced with an ever-growing list of unmet service and employment needs. Federal, state, and local governments are confronted with a downturn in the national economy after years of growth as well as with the heightened demand for homeland security. They are under enormous pressure to increase the provision of needed services while not raising taxes. Also rapidly changing the volunteer landscape is the decline of workers in the workforce. After peaking at nearly 30 percent in the 1970s the workforce growth rate is projected to drop 2 to 3 percent in the next ten years. Work and leisure will no longer be viewed as separate entities as older retired individuals cycle in and out of the workforce (Dychtwald et al., 2004). How do we respond to such demands in a way that will optimize scarce economic and human resources and develop cost-effective community service structures?

Clearly, new flexible and integrated models of work and service need to be pioneered. Organizations must develop new roles and paradigms of meaningful service opportunities. They must rethink and reframe their message of volunteerism in order to attract and retain a new generation of volunteers. They must integrate continuous best-practice methods with lifelong learning strategies, engage interdisciplinary, community, and collaborative partners, and employ market-driven strategies and incentives to harness untapped individual and community resources. It is time to move from policy proposals to action by actually creating and testing a variety of methods to achieve maximum engagement for current and future adults over age fifty.

Despite these known realities, organizations and society as a whole have been slow to embrace and apply many of the changes needed to attract a new generation of volunteer leaders. A number of emerging trends help illustrate a more clearly defined picture of individuals' expectations and needs concerning retirement and volunteerism.

- The number of seniors (sixty-plus) has doubled threefold since 1900. The senior population will double again by the year 2030 from 34 million to over 77 million.
- Increased longevity has resulted in more years of retirement and leisure time.
- There is a dearth of organized programs and policies that cater to meaningful life engagement beyond golf and shuffleboard (Morrow-Howell, Hinterlong, & Sherraden, 2001).
- Inefficient management of volunteer time is the number one reason individuals stop volunteering (two out of five—40 percent—have stopped volunteering for an organization at some time) (Treas, 1995).
- Forty-six percent of existing volunteers would volunteer more if meaningful service opportunities were readily available (Fleishmann-Hillard Research, 1998).

- Insufficient and inadequate outreach/practices by community organizations drive away volunteers in the fifty-plus age cohort.
- Many volunteer organizations lack effective infrastructure necessary to recruit and retain volunteers (Campbell, 2004).
- Retirees who have disengaged from the workforce have fewer formal and informal social networks that would increase the likelihood of volunteerism.
- Part-time retired workers may be more likely to engage in meaningful volunteer service opportunities (Herzog & Morgan, 1993).
- Adverse, negative stereotypes and labeling of older persons exist.
- A generalized lethargy or apathy among volunteer-based organizations to protect the status quo exists.
- Continuing education after retirement is an important part of meaningful life opportunities for the baby boomer generation (Hart, 2000).
- Volunteerism is not an integrated function or priority of the mission, staffing, or planning process of most service organizations (Campbell, 2004).

What emerges from this collage is a clearly identified set of problems and issues that compels us to rethink our traditionally held beliefs about retirement, older persons, active aging, motivations, and incentives for volunteerism and sustained community civic engagement. We can conclude then that the future generation of age fifty-plus volunteers will expect and demand more from their volunteer experience. They expect to be part of the decision-making process. They want flexibility that allows them to integrate paid and unpaid work. They seek engagement in meaningful opportunities similar to those offered to paid staff. They are motivated to transfer their professional skills to impact local community needs.

The university-based, lifelong learning and civic engagement Legacy Leadership Institute Model combines all of these elements into a single, flexible, and replicable model. This model promotes vitality for older adults and translates their skills, values, and expertise into meaningful, high-impact community service. Initially developed in 1998, the Legacy Leadership Institute Model has been adapted and implemented in multiple global settings since that time. It represents one example of the potential positive impact on business and communities alike in meeting both workforce and unmet human needs.

The Legacy Leadership Institute

Increased longevity in the United States and globally, combined with the pending retirement of the baby boom generation, have significantly heightened interest in the development of programs and resources that will be responsive to the needs, expectations, and desires of the fifty-plus population. One study indicates that 80 percent of baby boomers plan on continuing to work at least part-time after retirement (AARP/Roper, 2004). Other studies indicate that this group is more likely to volunteer as they will have additional leisure time. Herzog & Morgan (1993) conducted a survey among persons aged fifty-five-plus. Nearly 40 percent of nonvolunteers, the survey showed, would like to engage in some volunteer activity upon retirement. Recently, changes in the economy have made predictions less reliable regarding how the coming generations of fifty-plus persons will respond to work and leisure opportunities.

In addition, we know that there are several internal and external barriers that baby boomers and other younger retirees face when attempting to engage in meaningful community service. Those include

1. one's individual knowledge, perception, and motivation;
2. geographic barriers;
3. psychological barriers;
4. organizational barriers; and
5. the availability of resources.

Personal perception and motivation are principal factors in determining success in achieving meaningful, self-actualized roles in the community.

The university-based Legacy Leadership Institute Model was strategically designed to respond to the known needs and desires of the baby boomer generation and younger retirees. It provides a range of incentives and meaningful opportunities that result in the personalized application of acquired skills, enhanced learning, and community involvement. The Institute's mission is to prepare older persons to serve as multigenerational ambassadors who are committed to preserving the wisdom of the past, applying knowledge to community need in the present, and transferring these gifts to future generations. The Institute model serves to customize and deepen the individual level of community involvement in service activities through six broad goals:

1. Integration and utilization of the expertise of institutions of higher learning to create a visible, centralized base for the recruitment, training, and retention of volunteers aged fifty-plus.
2. Expansion of community capacity to meet unmet needs by creating a corps of well-trained fifty-plus volunteers who engage in community service through a university-based portal and who are committed to applying their time and talent to unmet needs.
3. Provision of greater flexibility and more service learning options for community involvement for volunteers that better match baby boomer expectations.
4. Development of a replicable, university-based infrastructure to attract, train, and coordinate a continuous stream of volunteers to fill a wide variety of community service needs.
5. Preparation and training for community-based organizations on designing and developing new approaches to working with baby boomer volunteers.
6. Development of evaluation standards and tools to measure the impact on volunteers and community organizations alike that would lead to national, state, and corporate policy changes.

Perception and motivation are central to the active engagement of the baby boomer generation. Boomers are highly motivated by opportunities set in the context of higher educational learning environments. Boomers are therefore likely to look to universities as a resource for increased knowledge, skills, and meaningful engagement. The Legacy Leadership Institute Model is the portal or entry point for boomers and younger retirees to engage in meaningful learning and active community service. Legacy Leadership students can customize their learning objectives and connect to active and sustained community service for personal and community impact.

The Legacy Leadership Institute Model emerged out of a series of demonstration projects designed to look at new ways to recruit and engage baby boomers in new or expanded volunteer roles. A series of focus groups with baby boomers helped to frame key issues which might affect baby boomer involvement in volunteerism. Several important issues emerged from those focus groups. First, baby boomers were not likely to become engaged with any program or opportunity that used words such as "senior" "older adult" or "retiree" in its description. Second, boomers associated the word "volunteer" as having low value or lesser status within the organization. The boomers stated that they would be more likely to volunteer if there were clearly identified roles which used their skills and abilities and offered an opportunity to learn new things.

The framework for the Legacy Leadership Institute concept was based on additional research and testing. Initially, the emphasis was on creating a recruitment and training structure that would appeal to baby boomers' priorities regarding future service (see Figure 6.1).

We have already presented substantiation of the boomers' high educational level and interest in continued learning. Findings have also been reflective of the need to develop meaningful volunteer roles that use the social capital, which boomers represent in effective ways. Finally, as adults begin to transition into partial or full retirement, they identify a need to replace the network of friends and colleagues with whom they shared goal-driven, work-related activities. They are looking for similar, goal-directed networks for their discretionary and service commitments. The Legacy Leadership Institutes are designed to incorporate all three priorities. A sixty- to eighty-hour classroom-

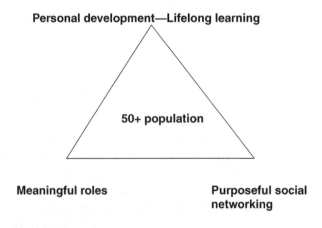

FIGURE 6.1. Theoretical basis for baby boomer involvement in Legacy Leadership.

structured curriculum provides the lifelong learning component. A collaboration with various community nonprofit agencies creates the opportunity to design meaningful volunteer roles. Ongoing meetings and learning activities among program graduates as a part of an alumni association provide a purposeful social network.

Once the initial Leadership Institutes were operational, it quickly became clear that there was another parallel set of structures and functions among nonprofit organizations that needed to be developed simultaneously if the graduating leaders were to have service opportunities which met their expectations. The baby boomers' personal needs intersected with needs from the nonprofit sector in this way (see Figure 6.2).

In order to put their extensive knowledge and newly acquired skills to work, the fifty-plus population would choose to volunteer in a nonprofit organization with a clearly defined and critical social mission. There is also a well-articulated need for a viable infrastructure that adequately supports not only paid staff but also unpaid staff. This infrastructure includes resources, access to management, training, job descriptions, recognition, and clearly defined roles in organizational hierarchy. Related to these factors are the needs for the nonprofits to

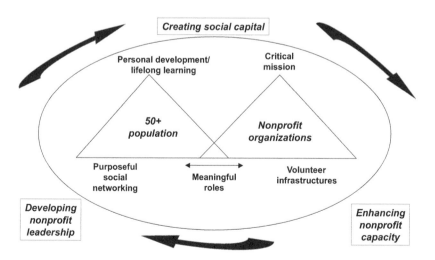

FIGURE 6.2. Theoretical basis for baby boomer involvement in Legacy Leadership. Legacy Leadership Model—University of Maryland, Center on Aging.

define roles for volunteers that are not only supported by infrastructure but also have personal and organizational relevance and meaning.

After returning from visits to nonprofits, the leaders returned to debriefing sessions to share their field experience and concerns about the ability of some organizations to fully utilize their potential. Despite having worked collaboratively with the nonprofits to define specific roles and offering several training sessions to nonprofit staff, leaders found that sustaining a meaningful volunteer role was not always easy. Although leaders were trained to work within existing organizational structures to make a difference, they sometimes reported feeling frustrated at the tendency of paid staff to revert to more "traditional" volunteer expectations and opportunities. In response, the newer iterations of Legacy Leadership Institutes contain training components for paid staff and formal opportunities for staff and legacy leaders to work together to define role expectations. The model for the program was then expanded. It became clear that in order to raise the professionalization of volunteering, not only must the future volunteers receive a broad knowledge base and clear role definition in a meaningful activity but paid staff must also receive training and assistance on working with baby boomer volunteers.

PROGRAM DESIGN AND STRUCTURE

The Legacy Institute Model is operationalized through the following six core components:

1. Program development and community partnerships
2. Recruitment and screening
3. Curriculum design and development
4. Volunteer leadership field placement
5. Graduation
6. Research and evaluation

Program Development and Community Partnerships

The Legacy Leadership Institute Model draws from and integrates the values, needs, and objectives of the local community. This goal is achieved by identifying key community informants from a broad spectrum of service and civic organizations to serve as an advisory steering committee providing direct input to the institute. This group is multidisciplinary and seeks out representatives from diverse organizations and other individuals to capture big-picture thinking. The advisory committee assists in identifying community needs and service gaps, assessing local best volunteer practices, proposing meaningful service opportunities for Legacy Leaders, identifying and securing local resources for sustainability, participating in team interviews for volunteer leaders, and providing input on select evaluation elements.

Each Legacy Leadership Institute focuses on a different segment of the nonprofit sector (e.g., health, literacy, environment) or on an unmet infrastructure need in the nonprofit organization (e.g., volunteer management, fund-raising, information systems/technology). The institute staff and advisory steering committee work in local communities to identify organizational partners who will work with Legacy Leaders. The institute staff seeks partners with the following characteristics:

- Demonstrated, innovative approaches to meeting identified needs in their community
- Ability to leverage and engage diverse community partners in service objectives
- Organizational profiles demonstrating sufficient managerial oversight and program integration
- Willingness to participate in project evaluation and research
- Responsive to articulated community needs
- Clearly defined scope of program objectives and ability to incorporate new volunteer objections
- Potential for ongoing collaboration
- Willingness to participate in a portion of classroom training and reflective sessions

Recruitment and Screening

A recruitment strategy to engage participants follows an intentional paradigm. Baby boomers are highly individualistic and thrive on new challenges and opportunities in which they can make a significant impact. The traditional "help wanted" shingle holds little meaning and appeal to the new generation of volunteers. Nonprofit agencies have already noted increasing difficulty recruiting volunteers over the age of fifty. New opportunities that use the time and talents of this cohort and effective marketing and recruitment approaches must be developed to attract potential volunteers. Prospective volunteers look for opportunities that will enhance self-development, bring personal life satisfaction, and create self-actualization of ideas and aspirations.

Considerable research has been done regarding perceived subliminal messages regarding advertisements and other marketing campaigns. Corporate slogans or business names are expressly chosen to convey a message that is internalized by the reader with the obvious intent of bonding the consumer to the product. The intent of the Legacy Leadership Institute is to attract a diverse group of participants and to create a marketing niche with broad appeal to the fifty-plus population. The feedback from accepted volunteer leadership students has confirmed the significance of selecting a strategic name. The word "leadership" attracted those who were seeking an opportunity to reengage in meaningful service in which they could apply their professional and personal skills. The word "institute" signified continuous learning, which is a strong core value for boomers. The word "legacy" resonated with their desire to choose activities with potentially high impact and lasting value.

Advertisements, as part of the process of recruiting leaders for the institutes, are placed in local newspapers as well as other venues such as libraries, the Internet, and with local employers. Lifelong learning opportunities and skills enhancement are emphasized. Nontraditional text such as "learn and gain new skills," "a unique opportunity," and "want to become involved in your community?" are utilized to attract the nontraditional prospective volunteer. The word "volunteer" is intentionally omitted from all materials in response to feedback that it implies "low-skill" activities. This approach has resulted in consistently attracting highly skilled, soon-to-be or recently retired participants, a trend not seen in more traditional, volunteer recruitment efforts. Volunteer recruits include retired CEOs, nurses, educators, marketing specialists, board members, military personnel, professional trainers, and mid-level managers from various corporate, governmental, and private sectors. Each Legacy Leadership Institute accepts a maximum of thirty participants with one to three classes per year.

The application process is intentionally designed to be competitive and mirrors that of applying for a professional, paid position.

Applicants call a designated phone number where program-specific information is provided. An initial telephone screening is conducted to ascertain the applicant's suitability for the program and to ensure their commitment to community service. Those who are successful at this stage are sent an application to complete. Applications are screened by staff for completeness and to determine who should be invited for a face-to-face interview. Successful applicants then participate in a team interview with staff and members of the leadership advisory committee. Subsequent program assessments have indicated that volunteer leadership students aged fifty-plus appreciated the intensive application and screening process, therefore professionalizing and adding value to the experience.

Accepted applicants must make a commitment to complete a minimum of 250-400 hours of combined lifelong learning and community service within a one-year period. Volunteer leaders usually work 8-10 hours per week with liberal allowance for vacations, caregiving, grandchildren, and other pursuits (see Figure 6.3).

Curriculum Design and Development

The Legacy Leadership Institute Model engages volunteer leadership students in forty-five to sixty-five hours of classroom learning followed by an unpaid, supervised field placement in a community-based organization. The intensive integration of lifelong learning skills coupled with meaningful service opportunities produces a committed, long-term volunteer who is more likely to engage in sustained civic activities. Volunteers who are highly knowledgeable concerning community resources, who have a good sense of their own self-worth, and who understand the dynamics of volunteerism are more likely to make an ongoing, volunteer commitment to communities.

The intent of the curriculum is to be academically challenging, provide meaningful life-application skills, and create a forum for significant interaction that focuses on problem solving, knowledge of community resources, and self-development skills. All Legacy Lead-

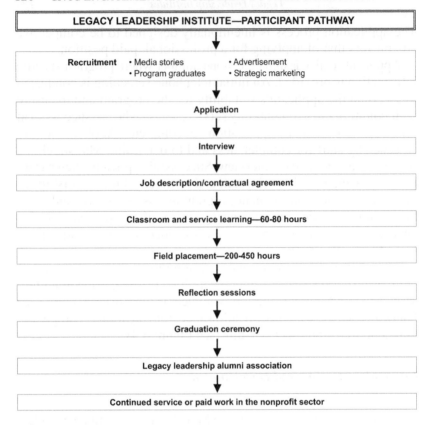

FIGURE 6.3. Theoretical framework for organizational involvement in Legacy Leadership.

ership students must complete the core curriculum. These courses are considered vital in understanding and transmitting a core knowledge base that can then be expanded and customized for individual pursuits. A matrix of subtracks is offered that allows them to engage in more personalized diverse learning environments and to learn new skills. This particular model is unique to the university setting. It effectively utilizes the vast resources of the university system while simultaneously partnering with community-based organizations to meet identified community needs. An overview of the program and model curriculum is shown in Figure 6.4.

| CORE CURRICULUM—ALL LEADERSHIP STUDENTS COMPLETE |

| Community networks | Volunteer leadership | Delivery systems |

- Demographic profiles
- Federal, state, and local policies
- Eligibility programs
- Need identification
- Program identification
- Community and civic organizations
- Navigating the system
- Agency/organization profiles

- Self-esteem and self-efficacy
- Communication skills
- Disengagement theories
- Role of volunteer leaders
- Team management
- Personal profiles
- New roles for volunteers
- Recruitment strategies
- Conflict resolution
- Transformational leadership

- Understanding paid and unpaid staff roles
- Organizational structures
- Cultural competence
- Volunteer? Where do I fit in?
- Service and community impacts
- Position descriptions
- Identifying system barriers
- Technology and volunteers

| ELECTIVE SPECIALTY SUBTRACKS FOR VOLUNTEER LEADERS |

- Volunteer coordination and management
- Intergenerational literacy
- Economic and workforce development
- Volunteer to work skills enhancement
- Humor skills programs for healthy living

- Public policy and social program development
- Fund-raising and development
- Environmental awareness and protection
- Health and independent living

| APPLICATION OF ACQUIRED KNOWLEDGE AND SKILLS IN COMMUNITY-BASED ORGANIZATIONS |
Site alternatives for community service

- Mediation and conflict resolution
- Humanitarian organizations
- Child and adult literacy programs

- Fire/rescue organizations
- Governmental and legislative offices

- Human service agencies
- Elementary, middle, or high schools
- Hospital and home health organizations
- Private sector firms
- Environmental programs

FIGURE 6.4. Legacy Leadership Institute curriculum.

Volunteers who have ongoing learning opportunities extend and deepen their contribution and commitment to sustained community service. The Legacy Leadership Institute Model encourages participants to assess and determine their own learning needs and to take an active role in planning and evaluating the learning experience.

Interactive learning techniques are employed to enhance the learning experience. Students often work in teams and with paid staff from nonprofits on creative problem-solving activities and other group exercises. These small group experiences create camaraderie among students and facilitate the importance of understanding different learning styles and the art of interpersonal negotiation. The Institute includes continuous exposure to knowledge about various community organizations and resources. This process occurs on two levels: (1) volunteer leadership students are advised of other community training opportunities and are encouraged to attend special conferences and seminars, and (2) representatives from community organizations are invited to make presentations about their programs during the course of the Institute. Site visits are made to select organizations to reinforce the classroom experience and provide a visual, interactive learning experience.

The Legacy Leadership Model is also unique in that co-learning opportunities are provided for paid staff from host organizations. A primary reason for the demise of many volunteer programs is the lack of staff acceptance and support. Staff members from our placement organizations have told us that the graduates of the Leadership Institute receive more intensive training and are better prepared for their assignment than their professional paid staff. The inclusion of paid staff in training programs at the Institute allows for simultaneous and integrated learning of both the volunteer leadership students and the paid staff of host organizations. This integration then reduces the tension between highly trained skilled volunteers and paid staff and facilitates a smooth transition for service collaboration.

Volunteer Leadership Field Placement

Providing volunteers with meaningful, supervised field placements is key to retention and high-quality service. It elevates, adds value, and professionalizes the volunteer experience. Legacy Leadership students are placed in teams of three or four at a particular site to reinforce the service-learning experience, create an esprit de corps, and leverage their collective expertise for high-impact service.

Each prospective placement site is screened by university staff to ensure sound internal operating practices and program policies that value and integrate volunteers. Approved service organizations must designate a direct supervisor, have preapproved position descriptions, actively engage volunteers in the decision-making structure of the agency, provide a variety of service learning opportunities, and afford volunteer leadership students opportunities for agency-wide participation.

Legacy Leadership students perform a host of sophisticated and multitask assignments such as drafting policies, research, fund-raising, and community development, outreach, public speaking, program development and implementation, information technology, volunteer management, facilitating child and adult literacy programs, and community relations. A university-supervised transitions coach is assigned to work with each student to assess the appropriateness of the match and to facilitate the communication process between the agency and the student.

Graduation

A graduation ceremony serves as the culmination point for the Legacy Leadership program. This highly visible event is attended by family members, host organizations, the media, institutions of higher learning, and invited national, state, and local representatives. Students who entered the program with little knowledge about community resources and civic engagement opportunities are now ready to make a sustained commitment to service.

Legacy Leadership graduates are then inducted into the Legacy Leadership Institute Alumni Association. The alumni association fosters continued, purposeful social networking, information sharing, informal support systems, and continuous lifelong learning training sessions. Inductees of the alumni association assist in future recruitment efforts and serve as peer educators for future volunteer leadership classes. Graduates are encouraged to continue their service and are retained in all longitudinal research studies (see Figure 6.5).

The Leadership Institute Model emerged out of a six-site demonstration project funded by the Corporation for National and Commu-

CIVIC ENGAGEMENT AND LIFELONG LEARNING MODELS
- ➢ Legacy Leadership Institute on Public Policy
- ➢ Legacy Leadership Institute on Nonprofit Fund-raising
- ➢ Legacy Leadership Institute on Humor Practices
- ➢ Legacy Leadership Institute on the Environment
- ➢ Legacy Corps for Health and Independent Living

COMMUNITY ADVISORY PANEL
- ➢ Assessment of community culture assets and needs
- ➢ Community collaboration

CORE LIFELONG LEARNING CURRICULUM
- ➢ Volunteerism
- ➢ Transformational leadership
- ➢ Nonprofit organizational structure and management
- ➢ Communication skills
- ➢ Community collaboration skills

SPECIALTY AREAS OF CONCENTRATION
- ➢ Public policy
- ➢ Community development and fund-raising
- ➢ Communications and humor practices to increase healthy lifestyle
- ➢ Conflict resolution and mediation
- ➢ Health and independent living
- ➢ Volunteer management
- ➢ Environment and environmental health
- ➢ Literacy

SKILLS DEVELOPMENT AND MENTORED PRACTICE
- ➢ Environmental educator
- ➢ Humor specialist in schools
- ➢ Literacy tutor
- ➢ Volunteer manager
- ➢ Fund-raiser
- ➢ Health education assistant
- ➢ Respite service assistant
- ➢ Mediator
- ➢ Legislative aide
- ➢ Personal care assistant

SUSTAINED CIVIC ENGAGEMENT
- ➢ Volunteerism
- ➢ Employment
- ➢ Community involvement

FIGURE 6.5. Legacy Leadership model overview.

nity Service and AARP from 1998 to 2002 and managed by the University of Maryland Center on Aging. Three of the six sites worked on developing variations of the model in their recruitment and retention for volunteer coordination, hospital to home assistance, and independent living service expansion.

The initial model, the Leadership Institute for Active Aging (Wilson & Steele, 2002), was developed in the site located in Palm Beach County, Florida. In its first three years, this site trained four classes of volunteer leaders for a total of 107 graduates. Those volunteers provided approximately 43,000 hours of service to over 7,200 individuals. Over 24,000 hours of service were direct service in respite care, medical insurance assistance, and literacy tutoring. Nearly 19,000 hours of indirect service were rendered in community organizing activities, crime prevention, marketing, public speaking, and intervention and prevention services. The financial impact was valued at $660,661. This figure was based on information obtained from the *Independent Sector* (2002) which calculates the hourly rate or value of time for a volunteer at $15.39 based on the average earnings of nonagricultural workers as determined by the U.S. Bureau of Labor Statistics. By the end of the fifth year of operation, this Leadership Institute produced 172,560 hours of service in the community valued at $2,500,000.

In the demonstration phase, the agencies in which Institute graduates were placed expressed high satisfaction with the quality, commitment, and capacities of those volunteers. In a written survey, 85 percent were either satisfied or very satisfied with their connection to the Institute. An ongoing assessment of service by graduates indicates that about 70 percent continue to serve in the community for an average of forty-six hours per month per person, a figure considerably higher than the eight to twelve hours per month currently identified as the average hours of service provided by older volunteers.

The University of Maryland Center on Aging began developing variations of the Leadership Institute Model that were relevant to community needs. This model, Legacy Leadership Institute on Public Policy (Wilson & Simson, 2002) sought to engage residents of Maryland over the age of fifty in volunteer service by first engaging them at the state level through training on public policy related to local and state policy issues and an internship with a government official during the ninety-day legislative session. The first class of twenty-five was chosen from over 200 inquires. This class was 60 percent male with a mean age of sixty-three. Prior to participation in the program, 24 percent had no involvement in volunteerism and 44 percent had volunteered an average of one to five hours per week. After graduation, 86 percent had plans for continued civic engagement including continued volunteerism in a legislative office, paid employment emerging from their Institute experience, or volunteerism based on an interest identified during their legislative placement. Since the initial public policy institute, a total of four classes of Legacy Leaders have been recruited and placed. More than half of the graduates remain actively engaged with the Legacy Leadership Institute for Public Policy as members of its steering committee, mentors to and recruiters of new leaders, speakers at Leadership Institute trainings, and as field placement supervisors. The majority of graduates participate in Legacy Leadership Institute Alumni Association networking activities. Although the Legacy Leadership Institute was initially created as a way to enhance civic engagement, changing economics have also caused it to serve as an avenue to achieve full- or part-time employment. Approximately 45 percent of participants are now employed, most in the nonprofit sector. Some were recruited to paid positions associated with their field placements or with the assistance of their site supervisors.

In 2004, after three classes had graduated, the program took two approaches to program sustainability. First, the program graduates worked with legislators to create a bill to provide permanent funding. Second, the graduates formed a leadership steering committee to continue the Institute primarily through volunteer assistance. Though the bill did not attain funding, the leaders continue to operate the Institute on a volunteer basis.

Three more Legacy Leadership Institute Models have recruited their second or third class of participants. The Legacy Leadership Institute for Nonprofit Fundraising initially was established in response to discussions with nonprofits who indicated the greatest unmet need they had in providing community service was in raising resources and funds for fiscal sustainability. A Legacy Leadership Institute was created to provide an opportunity for both nonprofit staff and volunteer teams to learn together and then to apply their knowledge to creation and implementation of a development plan. Early feedback indicates that there is a significant impact on the overall organizational infrastructure. As participants begin to develop their plans, the need for additional infrastructure, resource reallocation, and mission clarification identify areas on which to base funding requests. Numerous outcomes to date include the creation of new fund-raising committees and structures, the development of special events, and the creation of sponsorships.

Other Legacy Leadership Institute models have been created on environmental education and service and on healthy lifestyles for youths. These models were created in partnership with local environmental nonprofits and schools. They provide opportunities for more episodic service based on planned programs conducted periodically in which the Legacy Leaders play critical roles. In these as in all of the models, the Legacy Leaders are instrumental in shaping and refining the education and service elements of the Legacy Leadership Institute as well as helping with structural and functional changes to make the relationship with the nonprofit most effective.

RESEARCH AND EVALUATION FINDINGS ON THE LEGACY LEADERSHIP INSTITUTE MODEL

In developing new approaches to the recruitment, training, and retention of the next generation of volunteers, it was essential to assess the impact of the model on the leaders' nonprofit agencies and communities. All participants in the various iterations of the Legacy Leadership Institute concept are asked to participate in baseline and follow-up data collection. Participants training as leaders complete a baseline civic engagement instrument to assess their involvement to date in various civic and nonprofit sectors, paid and volunteer activities, and their self-rated health status. A modified version of this instrument is now being completed by LLI graduates on a yearly basis to determine ongoing changes in and intensity of their civic engagement and the potential role the LLI plays in that level of engagement. LLI participants, both volunteer and agency staff, complete baseline and follow-up assessments of their leadership self-efficacy. This research provides an important perspective on changes in perception on their ability to make a difference in the community and in the nonprofits in which they are placed for the field experience. Field placement supervisors are also asked to complete a leadership assessment instrument about their Legacy Leader in order to determine organizational perspective on the leadership role of the volunteer and how that perspective might change over time. Impact on the organizational structure of the nonprofit is determined by a baseline and follow-up instrument based on the Campbell (2004) study of volunteer management infrastructure in nonprofits and charitable organizations. Finally, impact measurements are defined for service goals for the various LLI models and measured with relevant baseline and posttest surveys.

The various iterations of the Legacy Leadership Institute Model were all designed around the core curriculum and framework that signifies this lifelong learning and civic engagement model. Each iteration provides opportunities for skills development and service that differ based upon the public sector and positions for which the LLI is providing preparation. The next section will provide selected findings from four of the 2003-2004 Institute participants. These measures represent the implementation of a more detailed evaluation model of comprehensive measures that will continue to be tracked over time.

Specific Findings to Date: Who Are the Participants?

The different models of Legacy Leadership provide skill development opportunities and service activities that are likely to attract differing types of participants into the programs. Although all Institute models include learning new skills, attitudes, and facts, the service activity related with each type of model is quite different. The LLI participants in this phase of the evaluation focused on environmental issues, fund-raising, and policy development activities with nonprofit organizations or legislative bodies.

The average age of LLI members is 59.9 years with a range from 30 to 78 years. The majority of LLI participants are white (70.3 percent). The LLI programs described here have no Hispanic participants but do report almost 14 percent who describe themselves as multiracial. Classes in 2004 recruited Hispanic participants. The LLI participants are a well-educated group with almost 45 percent reporting graduate or professional degrees (see Table 6.1). Almost half of the participants are married with more than 20 percent divorced and 13.5 percent separated. The LLI group is predominantly female but the Institute model attracts a larger concentration of male participants than does the direct service model of Legacy Corps for Health and Independent Living (described in Chapter 4). To date, the public policy institute has attracted a higher proportion of male participants than the other institutes.

Why Did the Members Join a Legacy Institute Program?

The Leadership Institute Model attracts members with varying and multiple motivations for joining. LLI members focused on expanding or utilizing their knowledge or skills (see Table 6.2). LLI participants appear to be interested in utilizing the Legacy Institute experience to explore future job opportunities or future paid employment. When asked to identify the single most important reason for joining, LLI members selected expanding knowledge and skills as the most important (24 percent) (see Table 6.3).

TABLE 6.1. Educational level of Legacy Leadership participants.

Educational category	Mean score
High school or equivalent	1.4
Vocational, some college	15.1
2+ years college	17.8
College graduate	20.5
Graduate/professional	45.2

TABLE 6.2. Reasons for joining Legacy activities.

Reasons	LLI percent
To expand knowledge or skills	86.0
To utilize my knowledge and skills	73.7
To explore future job or volunteer service opportunities	72.0
To help people or solve problems in community	64.9
To be involved in community	52.6
To join a network of others committed to community service	50.9
To work with people who have different backgrounds than I have	36.8
To eventually move into paid employment	24.6
As a moral obligation of my faith	15.8

TABLE 6.3. Most important reasons for joining Legacy programs.

Reasons	LLI percent	Rank
To expand knowledge and skills	24.0	1
To help people or solve problems in the community	16.0	2
To utilize my knowledge and skills	14.7	3
To be involved in community	14.7	4
To explore future job or volunteer service opportunities	8.0	5
To work with people who have different backgrounds than I have	2.7	6
To eventually move into paid employment	1.3	7

What Is the Relationship to the Home Community?

A scale was devised from five questions to measure participants' relationship to community. The assumption is that increasing commitment to one's community over time will lead to greater and longer-term commitment to volunteer activities. The five questions are as follows:

Q1: Do you feel that you make a contribution to the community?
Q2: Do you have a strong attachment to your community?
Q3: Do you have a good understanding of the needs and problems facing the community in which you serve?
Q4: Are you aware of what can be done to meet the important needs in your community?
Q5: Do you feel that you have the ability to make a difference in your community?

The scale devised from the five questions combines the responses from each of the individual probes, with higher scores representing stronger attachment to communities. At baseline, LLI participants report a cumulative score of 19.2. Variations do exist among the three types of institutes. The scores range from a high of 19.55 for the policy institute participants to a low of 17.86 for the environmental institute. However, this variation does not achieve statistical significance. Within institutes, variation does show interesting significant patterns for gender. Males within the different types of institutes score higher on the community attachment scale than females, with the larger differences noted in environmental and fund-raising activities (see Figure 6.6). No variations on this scale within the institutes were found on other demographic measures.

How Do Legacy Participants Participate in the Political Process?

A mark of civic engagement is the level of involvement in political activities. Scales of political activity have been utilized widely in political science literature and involve voting and other civic activities in which members might participate. The specific activities include, for example, voting in national or state and local elections, working for a candidate, attending rallies, writing letters to editors or legislators, working in a community organization that participates in advocacy, or starting community projects. The Civic Engagement Baseline Questionnaire included fourteen probes about political activities that members had been involved with prior to enrolling in Leadership Institute programs. The Likert-type responses were recoded into a scale of political involvement. The LLI participants report a substantially higher level of political involvement prior to joining Legacy Leadership than do participants in other types of direct service models around the country (see Chapter 4). The participants in the three

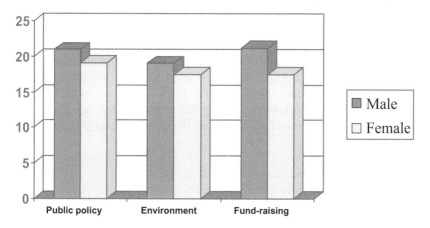

FIGURE 6.6. Community involvement scale by institute and gender.

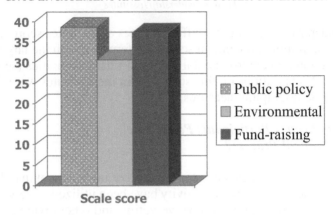

FIGURE 6.7. Involvement in political activities prior to Legacy participation.

types of institutes do vary significantly on this political participation measure. The public policy group reports an average scale score of 39.4 versus the lowest of the three from the environmental group at 30.7 (see Figure 6.7). The only demographic variable that influences variation between institutes and within institutes is educational level. Individuals with higher educational levels score significantly higher on the scale of political involvement.

How Do Members Expect to Be Involved After Legacy Training?

An important measure of success for Legacy models will be the impact that the training and volunteer experience has on members' decisions to continue to participate and be involved in their communities. Although longitudinal data will track their actual involvement over time, baseline data sought input as to the members' expected levels of involvement after completing the program. Six questions focused on expectations of involvement in specific types of activities.

Q1: How likely is it that you will be involved in community services in the future?
Q2: How likely is it that you will be a volunteer service leader in government?
Q3: How likely is it that you will be a volunteer service leader in a community organization (nongovernmental)?

Q4: How likely is it that you will participate in national service (e.g., foster grandparents, Peace Corps)?

Q5: How likely is it that you will work on a political campaign?

Q6: How likely is it that you will get involved in an organization that advocates specific policies?

The participants in the public policy institute report significantly higher expectations of future involvement in these types of activities, 34.1 compared to 31.2 for fund-raising participants and 20.3 for environmental participants (Figure 6.8). African-American participants in the institutes report highest levels of expectations for future involvement as do better-educated participants. These differences are statistically significant. LLI participants also represent new social capital or new resources in that 37 percent are new to the volunteer sector (have not volunteered before) and 35 percent have not performed caregiving activities (see Figure 6.9).

OUTCOMES AND CONCLUSION: THE IMPACT AND POTENTIAL OF THE LEGACY LEADERSHIP INSTITUTE CONCEPT

Findings indicate that the Legacy Leadership Institute Model is able to attract baby boomers and those near baby boomer age, the

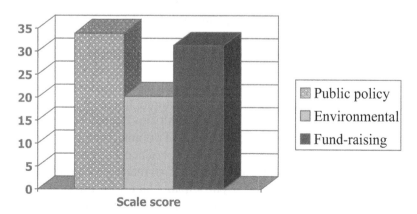

FIGURE 6.8. Scale comparisons of expected level of future involvement for Legacy participants.

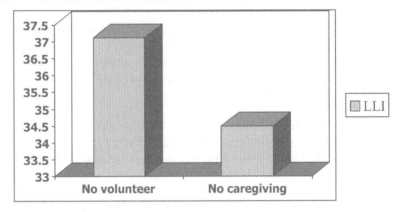

FIGURE 6.9. Involvement in volunteer activities prior to Legacy experience.

highly educated, and participants diverse in both gender and ethnicity. Although each institute tends to attract a slightly different configuration of Legacy Leaders, their profiles are similar to the baby boomer demographics, and individuals who might not otherwise have found a satisfactory entry point into making a personal commitment to civic engagement are active participants. Therefore, their expected level of future involvement with the community is quite high and follow-up data collection substantiates sustained levels of engagement with the community. The intent of the LLI models was to not only attract the fifty-plus population to participate but also to increase the potential of ongoing involvement at levels higher than current norms. To date, the model is fulfilling these expectations.

Process and outcome evaluations indicate that combining lifelong learning with civic engagement creates a powerful recruitment tool. Participants first entering into an LLI indicate that primary motives for attending are that the LLI was a structured, university-sponsored learning environment, and the opportunity to connect with others with a common purpose. The inclusion of volunteer community service as a part of the lifelong learning experience was not always the initial motivating factor in participation. Exit interviews with a subset of participants indicate that if participants had been informed only about the community service opportunities and the need for volunteers that most would not have been interested. The integration of a continuous, lifelong learning component that extends beyond the LLI classroom experience has broad appeal to younger retirees and to the baby boomer generation. Participants appreciated understanding the issues surrounding and the context in which their assistance might be valuable. Legacy Leaders stated that if the initial advertisement had focused solely on recruitment of volunteers that they would not have responded.

The lifelong learning and civic engagement model described here has broad organizational and community application. The strength of the model is its flexibility and adaptability to specialized community need and a variety of sectors within the nonprofit community. The two concepts of lifelong learning and civic engagement are building blocks for attracting and retaining a new generation of volunteers. This model offers organizations the opportunity to reframe their message, rethink their programs and services, and create a marketing niche through a partnership with both universities and potential volunteers.

The findings provide support for the large-scale replication of this model. Legacy leader models have expanded into multiple U.S. and global sites, a testimony to its adaptability to community need regardless of geographic locale and to its global resonance with the cohort to which it is targeted.

The interest in lifelong learning is not likely to diminish as the baby boomers age, but rather to increase. This interest provides a natural opportunity for colleges and universities to step forward and play a critical role in the ongoing active engagement of boomers by serving as a gateway to innovative and proven methods for entry into the community. The integration and utilization of institutions of higher learning to create a visible and centralized base for recruiting and training volunteers over the age of fifty is a seamless extension of the community service and service learning functions of the university of the twenty-first-century. It extends the applied learning aspects of the curriculum to older learners in a manner most appropriate and effective for this population. Concomitantly, the university, through the LLI, can use its knowledge and resources to expand the capacities of nonprofits. The cultural impact of the Legacy Leadership model is that of an additional avenue for the creation of an enhanced societal perspective on the capacity of the fifty-plus population through the development of substantive, new volunteer roles. The Legacy Leadership Model only offers a framework and tools to leverage the resources of younger retirees and baby boomers in volunteer positions but also in paid work in nonprofits.

Most baby boomers report the need or desire to continue to work after age sixty-five. They are, however, motivated to apply their knowledge and experience to new arenas, particularly to the non-profit sector in order to make a difference in their communities. The Legacy models have increasingly been adapted in order to serve this need. Legacy Leaders get training and practical experience in a new role as a volunteer and learn to understand the needs and structure of nonprofit agencies.

The future success of organizations seeking to access the vast capabilities of the next generation of fifty-plus volunteers will depend upon reassessing and thinking expansively and creatively about needs and service opportunities, strategically engaging other community collaborative partners, and employing market-driven strategies and incentives to attract and retain adequate numbers of volunteers. The Legacy models were developed in response to these needs and tested over a period of years to assess their effectiveness. Other innovations are being developed and there will be a need for even more approaches to be developed and implemented throughout the United States and globally if organizations are to be ready for the coming wave of potential talent and social capital represented by our aging society.

REFERENCES

AARP. (2004). *Baby Boomers Envision Their Retirement: An AARP Segmentaiton Analysis.* Washington, DC: AARP.

Campbell, K. H. (2004). *From Research to Action—A Unified National Response to the 2004 Volunteer Management Capacity Study.* Washington, DC: National Human Services Assembly.

Dychtwald, K., Erickson, T., & Morrison, B. (2004). *It's Time to Retire Retirement.* Harvard Business Review Product #R0403C. Boston, MA: Harvard Business School Publishing.

Fleishman-Hillard Research. (1998). *Managing Volunteers.* St. Louis, MO: Fleishman-Hillard Research.

Hart, P. (2000). *Retirement Redefined.* Washington, DC: Peter Hart Associates, Inc.

Herzog, A. & Morgan, J. N. (1993). *Formal Volunteer Work Among Older Americans.* Westport, CT: Auburn House.

Independent Sector. (2002). *Giving and Volunteering in the United States.* Washington, DC: Independent Sector.

Keefe, S. (2001). *Tapping Senior Power—Community Partnerships that Work.* Washington, DC: Corporation for National Service.

Morrow-Howell, N., Hinterlong, J., & Sherraden, M. (Eds.). (2001). *Productive Aging: Concepts and Challenges.* Baltimore, MD: Johns Hopkins University Press.

Treas, J. (1995). Older Americans in the 1990s and Beyond. *Population Bulletin,* 50(2).

Wilson, L. B. & Steel, J. (2002). *Leadership Institute for Active Aging.* West Palm Beach, FL: Area Agency on Aging of Palm Beach/Treasure Coast, Inc.

Chapter 7

An International Application of Lifelong Learning and Civic Engagement

Ben H. Slijkhuis
Joke M. Zwart

The Netherlands Platform Older People and Europe (NPOE) is a small NGO in the Netherlands that provides innovation in the (Dutch) older peoples' sector by looking at developments and best practices abroad. In 2001, the NPOE connected with the United States Legacy Leadership Institute of the University of Maryland Center on Aging that had set up courses for the new generation of seniors to become engaged in the voluntary sector. Since this American concept seemed to provide answers to some developments in the Netherlands, the two organizations decided to work together on establishing a similar concept in the Netherlands.

CORE ELEMENTS OF THE U.S. LEGACY LEADERSHIP CONCEPT

The situation in the Netherlands is very different from that in the United States and required a different approach. It was important to start by determining the core elements of the U.S. Legacy Leadership Institute. These elements would have to be taken over and embedded in a new approach that would fit the Dutch situation. The U.S. Legacy Leadership Institute is a university-based programmatic framework that utilizes the time and talents of volunteers age fifty and over and trains them for meaningful roles and civic engagement. The program offers sixty-four hours of instructional sessions on government, public policy, volunteerism, and leadership followed by field work experience in legislative offices

TRANSLATING THE AMERICAN CONCEPT
TO THE DUTCH SITUATION

The Netherlands is a country with a long tradition of volunteering. This country is among those with the largest volunteer involvement in the world (Salamon & Sokolowski, 2001). A Dutch study carried out in 2002 shows that 47 percent of all voluntary work in the Netherlands is carried out by people between fifty-five and eighty years of age (Knulst & Van Eijck, 2002). Our need was not only to involve more older people in volunteerism but also to involve a specific group of older people. Studies on the profile of the Dutch volunteer have shown that the baby boomer generation, those between forty-five and sixty years of age, are less active as volunteers (Knulst & Van Eijck, 2002). The average retirement age is relatively low in the Netherlands. The better-educated seniors are underrepresented in the voluntary sector. It is customary among people with high corporate positions to opt for early retirement in their mid- to late fifties. As a result, there is a large resource of people with knowledge and experience from which the voluntary sector could benefit.

The Dutch voluntary sector, although extensive and well-organized, faces a number of challenges. The nonprofit sector in the Netherlands is being challenged by changes in society. The Dutch central government is withdrawing financial support for nonprofit organizations. Because of a combination of work and caregiving, people have less time to devote to voluntary work and are becoming more discriminating as to what they do in their spare time. This applies particularly to the baby boomer generation. Boomers are often "sandwiched" between older parents and grandchildren for which they need to provide care, often in combination with their own paid job. A recent Dutch study about civil participation by older people shows that even though older people have more free time than younger people, they are being pressured in their free time to increase their labor participation. Older people in 2000 were more busy than those in 1980 and 1990 (Breedveld, De Klerk, & De Hart, 2004). The current government policy that actively promotes labor participation by older workers will put more stress on the voluntary participation of senior citizens in the future.

Voluntary work generally has a low status and society is becoming more and more individualistic, causing people to choose to spend their free time on themselves or with those in their immediate surroundings rather than for an organization to which they feel less commitment. These factors make it difficult for organizations to find new volunteers and to safeguard their continuity. Society as a whole is becoming more critical toward voluntary organizations, often demanding a more professional level of service. Due to government regulations and the economic situation in the Netherlands, certain sectors rely heavily on the help of volunteers, such as the health care and child care sectors. All of these factors exert much pressure on voluntary organizations and on volunteers themselves.

Other common problems within voluntary organizations are cooperation between professional staff and volunteers, and a lack of understanding between the board and the volunteers doing the actual work. Organizations often lack a policy on volunteer management that describes how to recruit, motivate, and support their volunteers. These factors call for organizational changes for which the organizations themselves are not always equipped. Voluntary organizations often lack the resources to hire professional interim managers or management consultants and rely heavily on the help of their volunteers who often lack the time or experience to find answers to the challenges their organization is facing.

These developments were taken into account when translating the American model to the Dutch situation. It was soon concluded that the Dutch voluntary sector was lacking volunteers with the kind of knowledge and experience needed to face these challenges. A plan was developed to try to attract volunteers who had fulfilled a career as professional managers in the corporate sector. This group typically did not enter the voluntary sector except, perhaps, in a board position. Therefore, the key questions we wanted to solve became: How do we attract retired senior managers from the corporate world to volunteerism and how can we use their knowledge and experience to strengthen the voluntary sector? It was clear that new voluntary roles needed to be developed for this group.

The answer seemed to lie in a similar approach that was used by the U.S. Legacy Leadership Institute. With our specific target group in mind, a course needed to be developed that would appeal to this group. Voluntary roles needed to be created that would offer them a new challenge while at the same time serving the struggling voluntary sector. The idea for the Senioren en Samenleving (SESAM)

Academy was born; an academic level course would be offered and graduates would become certified but voluntary consultants.

We also had to find the right terminology in translating the American model to the Dutch situation. Literal translation of the terms used in the American situation often resulted in a misconception of what was to be achieved. For example, contrary to the U.S. situation, the term "leadership" has a negative connotation in the Netherlands and needed to be avoided. "Making a difference," a term widely used in the United States, would also not work in the Dutch situation and was replaced by "contributing." "Community service" is an American concept for which there is no Dutch equivalent.

CONSTRUCTION OF THE DUTCH MODEL

In constructing the SESAM Academy we started with determining the output. The needs of the voluntary sector that we described earlier were used as a starting point. In order to ensure that our model would have added value, we had to ensure its output would be desired. We aimed at attracting retired managers from the corporate world, thereby providing the voluntary sector with an opportunity to benefit from a level of expertise that was normally not available to them. In order to appeal to this specific group, we decided to offer a high-quality program on an academic level.

Because our aim was to offer a program that was free of charge for the participants, it was vital that we find enough funding for the development and implementation of the SESAM Academy. A "committee of recommendation" consisting of a number of CEOs and ministers was established to attract corporate sponsors. Content development was assumed by an advisory council comprised of a number of experts, representatives from the voluntary sector, professional trainers, and researchers. These committees enabled us to stimulate cooperation between the voluntary and educational sectors as well as to base our model on a strong theoretical background. The committee of recommendation and advisory council worked closely with the project leader and trainer on the development of the course and on fund-raising. Meanwhile, we identified a central and tasteful location where the courses would be held that would appeal to the target group and sponsors. Recruitment of participants was started in the fall of

2002 with the help of sponsoring corporations. Since the concept was very new, we succeeded in obtaining a lot of free publicity.

THE SESAM ACADEMY

The Dutch model was named SESAM Academy. SESAM is an acronym for "Senioren en Samenleving" (seniors and society). The "academy" consists of a twelve-week course in which we build on the expertise and knowledge of the participants. This is an important aspect as it matches the way the baby boomers want to be approached. They seek to continue to develop themselves on a personal level after retirement while at the same time making use of the skills and experiences acquired during working life. The SESAM Academy offers such an opportunity. Although the term "leadership" was not used, the academy has a high focus on leadership.

During the twelve-week course participants attend two days of class per week. One day focuses on acquiring new skills such as advising or coaching, or new knowledge such as information on the culture of volunteer organizations. On the other day, one or two guest lecturers are invited to discuss issues that they encounter in their specific sectors or organizations. At the end of the course each participant takes on a three-week practice assignment that matches him or her with a voluntary organization. These experiences are discussed with other participants in class so that they can learn from one another and form clear pictures of their own specific interest areas.

Upon completion of the course, participants are awarded certificates during an official graduation ceremony. During the following year participants commit themselves to a number of hours of voluntary contribution as away to "pay back" for the free-of-charge course.

After retirement most participants lose professional networks. The SESAM Academy provides them with a new network of people with similar backgrounds and interests, and thus, the social aspect of the model is very important. Graduates of the SESAM Academy are able to stay in touch after the course through an alumni association. Many of them also stay actively involved as advisors in the academy itself, which, as a new organization, is still very much in the developmental phase.

THE RESULTS OF TWO YEARS OF SESAM ACADEMY

The SESAM Academy started with its first course in January 2003. In the first year, a total of fifty-seven SESAM advisors and coaches graduated. The corporate sector has responded postitively; many corporations include the SESAM Academy in the human resource policy for retiring senior management. The number of applicants so far has been overwhelming. In spring 2005 courses were not offered so that the semester could be used to create more connections with voluntary organizations for possible assignments.

MOVING ON: OTHER COUNTRIES ARE WAITING

The U.S. Legacy Leadership Institute and the Netherlands Platform Older People and Europe are now looking for ways to expand the concept of a training course aimed at the enhancement of voluntary participation by seniors across the U.S. and Dutch borders. The ideas, the experience, and the enthusiasm are there. Several contacts have been established with institutions in other European countries such as Germany, Ireland, Austria, Spain, and Slovenia. Together, this network is currently applying for European funding to set up a network of senior educators. This network would develop a general European framework that could serve as a basis for similar curricula in other European countries.

REFERENCES

Breedveld, K., De Klerk, M., & De Hart, J. (2004). *Ouderen en maatschappelijke inzet.* Den Haag, the Netherlands: Sociaal en Cultureel Planbureau for the Raad voor Maatschappelijke Ontwikkeling.

Knulst, W. & Van Eijck, C. (2002). *Vrijwilligers in soorten en maten II. Ontwikkelingen over de periode 1985-2000.* Tilburg, the Netherlands: University of Tilburg.

Salamon, L.M. & Sokolowski, W. (2001). *Volunteering in cross-national perspective: Evidence from 24 countries.* Baltimore, MD: The Johns Hopkins Center for Civil Society Studies.

PART IV:
INTERGENERATIONAL CONCEPTS
AND APPLICATIONS

Chapter 8

Intergenerational Relationships and Civic Engagement

Sally Newman
Richard Goff

INTRODUCTION

The post–World War II period in the United States has been characterized by two related demographic and social trends. First, the United States is aging. Since 1950, the median age in the United States has increased from thirty to thirty-four years and it is anticipated that it will continue to increase to forty-three by the year 2050. Moreover, the average life expectancy among Americans has steadily increased from 65.6 for men and 73.3 for women in 1950 to 74.0 for men and 79.6 for women in the year 2000. Second, the post–World War II period experienced a rise and subsequent decline of civic participation. The decline has a distinct generational flavor, as older people, who were civically engaged as young people, have maintained a high level of participation in civic organizations throughout their lifetime, while their younger counterparts demonstrate significantly lower participation rates (Putnam, 2000).

These trends are clearly interrelated and have profound social implications. Older people today are living longer, have more free time, and are healthier than their predecessors. Men and women born between 1910 and 1940 comprise what Robert Putnam refers to as the long civic generation who have participated in civic affairs throughout their lives (Putnam, 2000). This "civic minded" cohort is also concerned about the "traditional" family, the increase in single-parent households, and increased disconnection and disaffection of the young.

Civic engagement is a valuable social resource and is predicated upon the notion that voluntary collective activities strengthen community bonds and help to contribute to a strong democratic ethos. *Intergenerational civic engagement* can be defined as activities that include ongoing, purposeful interaction between older adults, children, and youths, and an exchange of resources and learning that meet the needs and enhance the quality of life of these generations. Typically, intergenerational exchange occurs between "skipped" generations of persons that reflect diverse educational, social, economic, and cultural backgrounds. The social and developmental needs of the elderly served by such programs include: the need to be productive, to be valued, to continue learning, to enhance their economic situation, to maximize their functionality, and to leave a legacy to the younger generation. In a complementary fashion, the social and developmental needs of youths involved in intergenerational programs are: to be cared for, to be mentored, to feel part of a community, to learn, to gain a historical perspective, to feel valued, to be educated, and to function effectively within the community and the family.

INTERGENERATIONAL CIVIC ENGAGEMENT AND SOCIETAL CONDITIONS

Recent social trends have prompted the development of intergenerational civic engagement models as a response to social issues. One of the most dominant social trends is the "normalization" of the nuclear family. Since 1945, the two-parent household living in a single-family dwelling unit has become the dominant and most socially recognized family structure. Often referred to as the "traditional" family, the *"Leave It to Beaver"* ideal is itself a relatively recent phenomenon. It is a product of post–World War II trends such as suburbanization, the advent and widespread use of modern household appliances, and the increased geographic mobility of families. Although *Leave It to Beaver* was not a documentary, these post–World War II social changes have produced families in which the elders and other extended family members are often absent, and sometimes living in other parts of the country (Coontz, 1992).

However, just as the nuclear family became the "normal" family model for many Americans, further social change undermined this family structure and is continuing to alter familial relationships.

Since the 1970s, there has been a marked increase in divorce rates and out-of-wedlock births. These trends, often associated with the so-called "crisis of the family," have contributed to further atomization of the family unit and the breakdown of extended, multigenerational familial relations.

The restructuring of the family is also connected to increased economic stress through shifting economic trends. Since the 1970s, families have experienced downward pressure on individual incomes inducing families to shift from sole-breadwinner arrangements to multiple-wage-earner situations. These situations often require the use of child care (either through daycare or through informal arrangements), which adds stress to the family structure and resources. Contributing to this stress has been the retraction of social spending from, e.g., Aid to Dependent Children, general assistance, and other aspects of the welfare state designed to help the family.

The net result is that the family unit, as it is conventionally conceived, has been finding it increasingly difficult to provide its traditional function. Traditionally, families provide social support, financial aid, mentorship, a sense of history and community, and are bridges between the individual and society. Without access to these resources, those most vulnerable and in the need of social support, often the young and old, find themselves isolated, without guidance, and lacking in basic social needs. Thus, the notion of *intergenerational programs* has emerged. These programs are designed to bring nonbiologically related individuals of different age cohorts together to share resources and services once performed by the family (Hanks & Ponzetti, 2005).

PROFILES OF YOUTH AND OLDER ADULTS AND IMPLICATIONS FOR INTERGENERATIONAL ACTIVITIES

The growing age stratification of the United States has corresponded with the cultural diversification of the United States. Both the younger and older populations in the United States display a significant level of diversity in cultural backgrounds, social influences, individual development, and individual needs. This section will address, in general terms, the characteristics of the United States elderly and youths with an understanding that the communities which engage in intergenerational civic programs will be drawing from the young and old of their community.

Older people, as a percentage of the U.S. total population, have tripled in number since 1900 and the median age in the United States (35.3 years) is as high as it has ever been in U.S. history. It is projected that the number of people in the United States, age fifty-five and older, will continue to grow to 66 million by the year 2030. Moreover, the number of old-old, that is people over eighty-five, will consist of 25 percent of those over 65 by 2050 (Hoyer and Roodin, 2003).

These changes in life expectancy are not uniform by race or gender. Typically, whites live an average of six years longer than African Americans with both groups experiencing a steady increase in life expectancy. Women outnumber men in older age cohorts. Women begin to outnumber men at the age of twenty-five and continue to outnumber in older groups. By age seventy-five, 61 percent are female and by eighty-five, 70 percent are female.

The term "older adult" or "senior citizen" includes people over sixty years of age and embraces several generations (Administration on Aging, 1965). With the increase in life expectancy, the age range of the "old" is significantly larger than previously experienced. One could argue that older adults are a multigenerational group in and of themselves. Given the diversity within this population, it is important to understand their capacities and limitations. Many elderly are categorized as "high functioning." They are relatively independent, free of major health problems, can hold down jobs, take care of themselves, and even take care of others. This group is most likely to be living on its own, with a spouse, or in senior housing that allows for the maximum independence of its residents. Though high-functioning older persons are present in all age groups, they are most concentrated within the fifty-five- to seventy-five-year-old group. This population contributes the largest number of participants in intergenerational civic engagement programs. Participants are drawn from the 58 percent of this cohort that are completely retired and the 23 percent that are retired but still working part-time (NCOA, 2002).

At the other end of the age spectrum, typically those over age eighty, many persons are lower functioning, dependent, and frail. They are more likely to have chronic illnesses or conditions that limit their mobility or vitality and which require partial or constant care from medical professionals. This group is more likely to live in residential housing that provides medical care, food, and social services to enhance the quality of their lives. This cohort is typically involved in civic engagement programs in which the young help the older adults. Across the age spectrum of the older generation that ranges from age sixty to over ninety, diverse levels of functionality are evident. There are many opportunities for people in this age cohort to participate in activities that demonstrate intergenerational civic engagement.

Similar to older persons, children are also a diverse group facing numerous social problems as a result of changes in our society. There are over 72 million children in the United States, including 23 million preschoolers and 49 million school-age children. Despite the fact that the United States is the wealthiest nation on the earth, nearly one in five children live in poverty. Those most likely to live in poverty are the youngest (under age six) (Children's Defense Fund, 2002).

Many of the recent social trends, which have contributed to popular debate around the "crisis of the family," have fallen on the shoulders of children. The number of children being raised in homes with working mothers increased from 38 percent in 1975 to 61 percent in 1999. Currently, one-third of all children born in the United States have parents who are not married. Children adopted from foster care increased to a record high of 45,821 in 1999. In addition, 2.4 million grandparents are recorded as the primary caregivers for their grandchildren. Nearly 20 percent of caregivers and their grandchildren are living in poverty (Children's Defense Fund, 2002).

In our current society, many "traditional" families are finding themselves increasingly strained to provide adequate financial support and care for their children. In nontraditional families, such as households in which one or both biological parents are absent, families face additional burdens. The limited level of public assistance available to families compounds the problems that children face. According to the Children's Defense Fund, no state pays enough cash-assistance benefits for a family to live on. In addition, 9.2 million children (almost one in eight) have no form of health insurance.

As children get older, arranging childcare for school-age children during nonschool hours can be a significant problem for many households. The ages of six to twelve are a time of significant emotional and developmental change. According to one recent study, children ages six to twelve are at risk of physical injury, emotional and psychological harm, and poor physical, social, and intellectual development if they have unstructured hours lacking supervision (Capizzano, Tout, & Adams, 2000). As a solution to this problem, approximately 40 percent of families with working mothers use "enrichment activities" or similar forms of supervised care during nonschool hours while the parents are working. The teen years are historically the time for preparation for work or college. However, within the past decade data on high school drop-out rates, teenage pregnancy, and teenage unemployment alert us to a large number of youths who are not preparing for a productive future. The Children's Defense Fund (2002) has reported that between 1997 and 1999 one in seven high school students dropped out of school, one in eight between sixteen and nineteen years of age were unemployed, and about one in ten became teenage parents.

Though this section has presented examples of children and youths for whom intergenerational civic engagement experiences would be of particular value, it is important to note that the concept of intergenerational exchange has intrinsic worth for *young and old* across the socioeconomic, educational, and ethnic spectrum of our society.

INTERGENERATIONAL MODELS IN THE UNITED STATES

Fundamental to the development of intergenerational programs as civic engagement models are the mutual benefits derived by the young and old participants. The level and type of benefits are a function of program components, intergenerational interactions, roles of the participants, degree of personal and group collaboration, strengths each group brings to the program, and the relationships that develop between the young and old. Intergenerational civic engagement can be divided into four models:

1. Older adults help children and youths.
2. Children and youths help older adults.
3. Children/youths and older adults help one another.
4. Children/youths and older adults help the community.

Since the 1980s, there has been a plethora of intergenerational programs (IPs) in the United States with an estimated several million participants (Generations United, 2002). They are visible in cities, suburbs, and rural communities. The young participants include average, gifted, and special-needs children and youths from two to twenty-one years of age. The older adults are represented by persons aged fifty-five to the late nineties who range from high functioning and independent to dependent and frail. Within the various intergenerational program models, different age cohorts alternate as service providers and service recipients. The roles and benefits for each generation shift as the participants alternate between provider and recipient. Irrespective of their roles, both generations experience the benefits of the intergenerational exchange. These models are detailed as follows.

Model 1: Older Adults Help Children and Youths

Older adults serve as tutors, mentors, coaches, teachers, nurturers, role models, and special friends to children and youths ages two to twenty-one. Programs are being implemented in a variety of environments including early childhood centers, schools, libraries, art centers, museums, universities, early childhood, family, and community centers or the homes of individuals. Older adults interact with individuals and small groups of young people. The interactions are designed to support the development of academic, social, and self-management skills of the young. In many of these models older adults receive training to enhance the effectiveness of these interactions (Newman, Ward, Smith, Wilson, & McCrea, 1997).

Model 2: Children and Youths Help Older Adults

Children and youths serve as visitors, guides, mentors, entertainers, tutors, and friends to dependent or frail older adults typically aged eighty to ninety plus. Many of these older persons are victims of Alzheimer's disease or other forms of dementia. This model is implemented in adult day-care centers, long-term care/residential environments, and in individual homes. The youths from ages four to twenty-one interact in groups in institutional settings or one-on-one in individual homes. The interactions are designed to improve cognitive and so-cialization skills, enhance activities of daily living, and to enrich the overall quality of life of frail elderly. The youths involved in these models are oriented to the needs of the older participants and engage in age- and skill-appropriate activities under the supervision of professional staff (Roth, 2004).

Model 3: Children/Youths and Older Adults Help One Another

A variety of intergenerational civic engagement models enable older adults, children, and youths to learn and grow together, helping one another to maximize their lives. Examples of this model are cross-age literacy programs in which old and young collaborate in language teaching/learning activities; in-service learning programs in which college students interact with and help older adults as part of their course work; and shared-site programs in which young children and the elderly share the same physical site for several hours daily and engage in planned and spontaneous supervised activities designed to promote cognitive, social, and physical development (Generations United, 2002; Newell & Beach, 2005).

Model 4: Children/Youths and Older Adults Help the Community

Communities in some regions of the United States involve young and old in team activities to enrich the lives of other community members. This model is an intergenerational civic engagement experience that involves individuals and organizations in which the larger community benefits directly from the collaboration. Teams of youths and older adults work together in various projects that benefit the community. They visit children and elderly in hospitals, residential care facilities, and at home. Youth organizations such as YWCA and YMCA and Boys & Girls Clubs team with senior citizen organizations involving community activities such as holiday events and fund-raising (Nichols, 2003).

THE STRUCTURE

As intergenerational civic engagement models increase in number interest has grown in learning about the structure of these models, the problems they confront, and their impact on participants and the communities in which they are being implemented. In the 1980s, evaluation and research initiatives began reporting on strategies for understanding, developing, and replicating successful intergenerational programs. Intergenerational programmers interested in the maintenance and replication of these models described characteristics that were indicators of success (Ward, Walson, Nicholson, & Newman, 1996). In an effort to replicate this success, training programs were developed with curricula materials focusing on characteristics to enhance successful development (Hawkins, Macguire, & Backman, 1999; Senior Service America, 2002).

Consistent with new information related to successful programs was a growing awareness within universities of the need to prepare students for jobs in human service fields in which intergenerational skills were desired. Texas Tech University developed an intergenerational curriculum specifically for youths interested in entering the field. The curriculum was introduced into secondary schools and community colleges and included skills appropriate to prepare students for entry-level intergenerational jobs in early childhood and aging areas (Texas Tech, 1994).

At another level, university trainers and researchers began to report on observable and measurable professional skills/competencies that were demonstrated by service providers in career-track positions. Managers and research observers noted the relationship between these skills and the success of intergenerational programs (Olson, 1994). Program-related professional competencies were identified and integrated to prepare students and professionals in human service fields for career-track work in intergenerational models (Senior Citizens America, 1998; Larkin & Newman, 2001).

Since the 1990s, university faculty have examined the relationship between intergenerational concepts and career application. They report links between practice and academic learning that could increase intergenerational knowledge and skills and promote professional career directions. Intergenerational civic engagement programs have become an area for multidisciplinary discussion because of their complex structure, academic implication, relevance to various social service fields, and potential impact on social change (Larkin & Newman, 1996; Kingson, Bowers, & Moore, 2002; Roodin, 2003; Roodin & Kraus, 2003).

As examples of intergenerational models continue to develop, standards and guidelines for practice have become essential. Currently, there is an initiative designed to establish a common knowledge base for unifying the intergenerational field with standards, and ensuring effective professional practices. The initial guidelines were disseminated for feedback, revised several times, and are being piloted in a graduate course at the University of Findlay (Rosebrook & Larkin, 2003).

The growth of intergenerational program initiatives during the past thirty years has caused an increase in the literature. Valerie Kuehne's book, *Intergenerational Programs: Understanding What We Have Created,* is timely and important and helps us move forward in the discussion of the intergenerational field. Kuehne presents an overview of the conceptual underpinnings and outcomes of intergenerational programs. She provides insights about the structure of IP models, aspects of intergenerational programming strategies, and the proposed future as a field of study and as a civic engagement model.

PROBLEMS AND CHALLENGES

Currently, intergenerational programs are striving to become a model for social change. This expectation brings with it problems and challenges. As social planning models these programs address the needs of the two populations at the opposite end of the human continuum and in so doing embrace the community at large. In order to meet the needs of these populations, IPs involve multiple systems that, because of different goals, constraints, funding sources, and advocates do not typically collaborate. However, to meet the needs of both generations, a new process for partnering will need to be established. This process will face the following challenges:

- How to link the current infrastructure of separate systems without sacrificing the uniqueness of each system
- How to prepare staff and administration whose focus is on one age cohort to understand and embrace the needs of multiple age cohorts

- How to motivate funding resources to value cross-age partnerships and social programs that can impact the larger community
- How to interest the community in the new partnerships and then validate the concept of intergenerational civic engagement as a viable approach to social change
- How to promote public policy initiatives that embrace the value of intergenerational civic engagement program models

To approach these challenges we refer to the recommendations of the 1996 national Johnson Foundation Wingspread Conference "Strengthening the Social Compact: An Intergenerational Strategy" that promulgated several intergenerational program management strategies designed to: impact intergenerational outcomes, support the ongoing development of best practices, and influence public policy in intergenerational civic engagement (Kingson, Gornman, & Leavitt, 1996).

The management strategies are grouped into three strategic directions. Subsumed within each strategy are recommended action steps that can be implemented by individuals and organizations and are directed toward the promotion of intergenerational relationships and civic engagement.

1. *Encourage citizen participation in communities.* The action steps recommended within this strategy include a variety of individual, community, corporate, and organizational activities that encourage infrastructure development and promote intergenerational initiatives in the social fabric of the community. Examples of action steps include: promote private/public/corporate partnerships that support community service initiatives; increase intergenerational initiatives on university campuses; increase community dialogue; and develop structures to encourage elders as community leaders.

2. *Strengthen the ties between generations through public policy.* The action steps recommended within this strategy establish the groundwork for the integration of intergenerational civic engagement into the public policy agenda at the local, state, and national levels. Examples of action steps include: advocate for collaborative intergenerational legislative agendas; define, pri-

oritize, and disseminate key intergenerational policy issues; develop coalitions and train intergenerational political activists.
3. *Promote the intergenerational vision.* The action steps recommended within this strategy focus on educating our society about the message, rationale, and importance of intergenerational initiatives. Examples of action steps include: clarify the message that intergenerational programs work; provide local organizations with assistance and ideas on how to promote intergenerational messages; and reframe the generational conflict message around the interdependence of generations.

BEST PRACTICES OF INTERGENERATIONAL MODELS

Intergenerational civic engagement initiatives are works in progress. This program planning model is slowly emerging as a vehicle to enhance social change and is currently being implemented in multiple human service venues. Though there is diversity among the program models, evaluation and research has provided information identifying consistent practices that result in successful programs. These practices are characteristic in programs that vary in size, population, goals, and projected outcomes. Best practice characteristics of intergenerational civic engagement programs include the following:

- Program benefits older and younger participants
- Program meets a defined community need
- Goals and objectives are clearly defined
- Collaboration exists between systems/agencies involved in the program's development
- Roles and responsibilities of participating professionals/volunteers are clearly defined
- Administrative and program staff are committed to the program
- Staff and volunteers are well-trained
- Staff is sensitive to the needs and expectations of the participants (young and old, professional and volunteer)
- Evaluation strategy is explicit as part of the program design and implementation
- Community support and involvement is integral to the program's development

OUTCOMES

Participant outcomes are typically reported in the context of impact on cohort groups and the development of personal intergenerational relationships. In this section we will highlight the impact of these models on young and old cohorts and will summarize information on intergenerational relationships that develop as an outcome of individual involvement. The information reflects program evaluations provided by participants, staff, outside evaluators, and researchers. Information is gathered from surveys, questionnaires, focus groups, logs, and observations.

IMPACT ON AGE COHORTS

Older Adults As Helpers

We have learned that intergenerational experiences such as mentoring, tutoring, nurturing, coaching, and serving as role models for children and youths contributes to the successful aging of independent, high-functioning older adults. These experiences enhance the self-confidence, skills, and feelings of self-worth of the older participants. In these models, older adults assume new and meaningful social roles in the community (Kuehne, 1992; Moody & Disch, 1989; Newman, Vasudev, & Onawola, 1985). When involved in program planning, older adults report an additional increase in their self-esteem and productivity (Dellman-Jenkins, 1997; Kocarnik & Ponzetti, 1999). Older adults' involvement in educational (school) settings with young people contributes to their own learning and memory and to a reaffirmation of worth. Their consistent presence in a learning involvement that stimulates cognitive development of children seems to also reinforce the cognitive functioning of older adult tutors (Newman, Karp, & Faux, 1995). Serving as caregivers for young children in nurturing and learning activities that enhance children's growth reinforces older adults' sense of self-worth, self-confidence, and contributes to life satisfaction (Newman, Larkin, Smith, & Nichols, 1999).

Young and Old As Partners

Partnerships between elderly and youths in programs that impact the community result in an increased understanding by both groups of the important role of all citizens (Kaplan, 1997). Intergenerational collaboration reinforces the feeling of empowerment of teams of young and old. This empowerment is a desired outcome of intergenerational civic engagement models. Undergirding program models involving older adults as helpers or providers of service is the concept of generativity as an important aspect in the stages of development for older adults (Erikson, 1950). In these programs older adults guide and care for younger persons They fulfill their own developmental needs, and transfer values, skills, and culture while contributing to the environment and the development of another generation (Kuehne, 2000; VanderVen, 1999).

The Young As Helpers

Evidence shows that there is an increase in physical well-being, cognitive functioning, and activities of daily living for frail older adults who interact with children and youths. Even persons with Alzheimer's disease and other forms of dementia become more responsive and engaged in the presence of children (Camp et al., 1997; Ward, Los Camp, & Newman, 1996). The isolated and lonely elderly interacting with youths as friendly visitors respond to the social stimulation and articulate a renewed sense of connection to the community.

Young and Old As Reciprocal Learners

Several program models exist in which youths and elderly help each other. From these programs we have information on learning outcomes for both cohorts. For example, in cross-age literacy models, both age groups report increased skills and an increase in pride and self-worth. Young and old as learners become comfortable with our language and culture and develop a feeling of belonging and acceptance (Power, 1998). In shared-site programs such as adult/child day care, community centers, senior housing facilities, schools, computer centers, long-term care centers, and planned neighborhoods both young and old report skill development, increased socialization, access to resources, motivation to learn, and a sense of belonging and acceptance (Generations United, 2002). College-age participants in intergenerational service learning programs interact with and help the community's older adults as part of their education. The college students and older adults report learning technical skills such as computers, and behavioral skills such as conflict and stress managment, especially in age-diverse environments (Hanks & Icenogel, 2001). Students reflect on increased understanding of the needs of dependent and independent older adults and develop and increase respect and understanding of this population's contribution to the community (Power, 1998). Older adults, similarly, describe a greater sensitivity to and understanding of the youths. Both groups report an awareness that their relationships contribute to an appreciation of the continuity of life.

Young As Helpers and Service Receivers

Multiple programs exist in which children and youths are involved with both independent and dependent elderly, as providers or recipients of service. When the youths are helped by older tutors, mentors, or care providers there is student improvement in academic and social skills, increased motivation to learn, changed behaviors, and an increase in self-esteem and self-worth (Newman & Larimer, 1995). For children in preschool and early childhood settings, teachers describe more cooperative behaviors, an ability to stay on task, and an increase in happiness. School-age youths and older teens report new insights about values, history, and culture. For children and youths who help the dependent elderly the data highlight the development of caregiving skills, an awareness and respect for the survival and self-management skills of the frail elderly, and an interest in aging as a field of study and work

INDIVIDUAL INTERGENERATIONAL RELATIONSHIPS

To date we have limited formal reporting on the relational impact of the intergenerational civic engagement experiences shared by old and young. Over the years parents, older adults, children, youths, professional caregivers, teachers, and faculty have informally commented on the experiences and the resulting relationships that evolve between the generations. Their comments reaffirm feelings that reflect positive human relationships. Reports received from focus groups, logs, letters, and quotes consistently include positive relational terms. They portray respect, trust, caring, friendship, concern, commitment, sharing, gratitude, happiness, remembering, and love and written or spoken expressions that give personal meaning to the relationships emerging from intergenerational exchange. Here are some of the feelings captured through representative quotes from program participants:

> Liz is like a breath of fresh air. She keeps me connected to the world of poetry I so love and to the community I can no longer see. (Quote from a blind eighty-year-old woman; former teacher whose seventeen-year-old weekly friendly visitor read Shakespeare to her and shared stories about the neighborhood. Their relationship was sustained for three years.)

> I really enjoy having an older person to talk to and to share part of my life with. This experience is great and helped me grow and understand more about myself today and when I grow old. (A teenage volunteer who visited the same two older adults in a retirement home for ten months.)

> We older adults have an awful lot to offer and gain. The children learn from us and we learn from them. I believe they really appreciate our compassion and love and they love us back. (Older adult caregiver in an early childhood center.)

> We older people are most apt to possess the qualifications children need most: love, time, dedication, and the willingness to learn. Many of us say, "If I can help a young person I pass along the way then my living will not have been in vain." (A tutor/mentor with fourth- and fifth-grade children.)

> I looked forward each week to helping an older adult immigrant learn our language and culture. I looked forward also to getting to know these brave, warm survivors filled with excitement and joy to be here and trying to fit in. They are great and I am privileged to be part of this program. (A college student participating in an intergenerational service learning course.)

CONCLUSION

The positive impact of intergenerational civic engagement program models on age cohorts and individuals is evident. As a policy phenomenon, we will need to examine the implications that can contribute to the development and maintenance of this social planning model. Generations United, the U.S. intergenerational advocacy organization, prepared a summary of legislative action during the 108th Congress that, if passed, would reinforce intergenerational civic engagement models. Their action priorities reflect recommendations in three overriding policy initiatives that can affect the quality of intergenerational civic engagement initiatives in the United States. Generations United

- recommends the support of community learning centers and intergenerational shared sites;
- encourages government resources to promote the Younger Americans Act that includes positive development of young people through intergenerational opportunities;
- recommends the reauthorization of the Corporation for National and Community Service and an increase in funding for the expansion of demonstration projects under the Senior Corps program;
- encourages restored funding for the social services block grant to its full level at $2.8 billion;
- supports raising the income threshold and lowering the age requirement for foster grandparents to make more senior volunteers eligible for the program;
- consistently publicized the importance of the LEGACY Bill that will provide access to safe affordable housing for grandparents and other relative-headed households;
- supports allocation of additional Fair Housing Initiatives Programs (FHIP); and
- encourages funds to grand-family education and a nationwide survey of the housing and service needs of grandparents and other relatives raising children.

The growing needs of our most vulnerable populations demand that we create a national climate in which all generations are integrally involved in the planning process for social change in the twenty-first century and in which the concept of civic engagement and quality of life for all generations become the national norm throughout the United States.

REFERENCES

Administration on Aging. (1965). *Older Americans Act.* Washington, DC: Administration on Aging.

Camp, C. J., Judge, K. S., Bye, C. A., Fox, K. M., Bowden, J., Bell, M., Valencic, K., & Mattern, J. M. (1997). An intergenerational program for persons with dementia using Montessori methods. *The Gerontologist,* 37(5): 688-692.

Capizzano, J., Tout, K., & Adams, G. (2000). *Child care patterns of school age children with employed mothers.* Washington, DC: Urban Institute.

Children's Defense Fund. (2002). *The state of children in America's union.* Washington, DC: Children's Defense Fund.

Coontz, S. (1992). *The way we never were: American families and the nostalgia trap.* New York: Basic Books.

Dellman-Jenkins, M. (1997). A senior-centered model of intergenerational programming with young children. *Journal of Applied Gerontology,* 16(4): 495-506.

Erikson, E. (1950). *Childhood and society.* New York: W. W. Norton.

Generations United. (2002). *Reaching across the ages: An action agenda to strengthen communities through intergenerational shared sites and shared resources.* Washington, DC: Generations United.

Hanks, R. S. & Icenogel, M. (2001). Preparing for an age-diverse workforce: Intergenerational service learning in social gerontology and business curricula. *Educational Gerontology,* 27(1): 49-71.

Hanks, R. & Ponzetti, J. (2005). Family studies and intergenerational studies: Intersections and opportunities. In Larkin, E., Friedlander, D., Newman, S., and Goff, R. (Eds.), *Intergenerational relationships: Conversations in practice and research across cultures* (pp. 5-22). Binghamton, NY: The Haworth Press.

Hawkins, M., McGuire, F. A., & Backman, K. F. (Eds.). (1999). *Preparing participants for intergenerational interaction: Training for success.* Binghamton, NY: The Haworth Press.

Hoyer, W. & Roodin, P. (2003). *Adult development and aging.* New York: McGraw Hill.

Kaplan, M. (1997). The benefits of intergenerational community service projects: Implications for promoting intergenerational unity, community activism and cultural continuity. In Brabazon, K. & Disch, R. (Eds.), *Intergenerational approaches in aging: Implications for education, policy, and practice* (pp. 211-218). Binghamton, NY: The Haworth Press.

Kingson, E. R., Bowers, A., & Moore, P. (2002). The intergenerational concept: Settlement houses without walls. Paper presented at GSA Meeting, Boston, November 22-26.

Kingson, E., Gornman, J., & Leavitt, J. K. (1996). *Strengthening the social compact: An intergenerational strategy 2000 and beyond, building an action plan for the intergenerational movement.* Pittsburgh, PA: Generations United.

Kocarnik, R. & Ponzetti, J. (1999). Corporate opportunities for intergenerational linkages: A human resource perspective. In Kuehne, V. (Ed.), *Intergenerational programs: Understanding what we have created* (pp. 149-160). Binghamton, NY: The Haworth Press.

Kuehne, V. S. (1992). Older adults in intergenerational programs: What are their experiences like? *Activities, Adaptation and Aging,* 16(4): 49-67.

Kuehne, V. S. (Ed.). (2000). *Intergenerational programs: Understanding what we have created.* Binghamton, NY: The Haworth Press.

Larkin, E. & Newman, S. (1996). Intergenerational studies: A multi-disciplinary field. *Journal of Gerontological Social Work,* 28(1-2): 5-16.

Larkin, E. & Newman, S. (2001). Benefits of intergenerational staffing in preschools. *Educational Gerontology,* 27(5): 2-15.

Moody, H. & Disch, R. (1989). Intergenerational programming between young and old. *The Generational Journal,* 1(3): 25-27.

National Council on the Aging, Inc. (2002). *American perceptions of the aging in the 21st century.* Washington, DC: NCOA/AARP.

Newell, D. & Beach, R. (2005, anticipated). Implementation and delivery of an intergenerational community learning experience. *Journal of Intergenerational Relationship,* 3(1).

Newman, S., Karp, E., & Faux, R. (1995). Everyday memory of older adults: The impact of intergenerational school volunteer programs. *Educational Gerontology,* 21: 569-580.

Newman, S. & Larimer, B. (1995). *Senior citizen school volunteer programs: Report on cumulative data.* Pittsburgh, PA: Generations Together.

Newman, S., Larkin, E., Smith, T., & Nichols, A. (1999). *To help somebody's child—older adults making a difference—Final report.* Pittsburgh, PA: Generations Together.

Newman, S., Vasudev, J., & Onawola, R. (1985). Older volunteers' perception of impacts of volunteering on their psychological well-being. *Journal of Applied Gerontology,* 4(2): 123-134.

Newman, S., Ward, C., Smith, T., Wilson, J., & McCrea, J. (1997). *Intergenerational programs: Past, present and future.* Washington, DC: Taylor and Francis.

Nichols, A. (2003). The Link Project: An intergenerational statewide collaborative project. *Journal of Intergenerational Relationships,* 1(2): 33-46.

Olson, S. L. (1994). *Competencies for intergenerational practice.* Stout, WI: University of Wisconsin.

Power, M. (1998). Aging in a metropolitan society. In McCrea, J., Nichols, A., & Newman, S. (Eds.), *Intergenerational service learning in gerontology: A compendium* (pp. 65-70). Pittsburgh, PA: Generations Together.

Putnam, R. (2000). *Bowling alone.* New York: Simon & Schuster.

Roodin, P. (2003). Developing administrative support and recognition for intergenerational service learning. Paper presented at the Annual Meeting of AGHE, St. Petersburg, Florida, March 6-9.

Roodin, P. A. & Kraus, C. R. (2003). Intergenerational service learning outcomes: Developing a research agenda for the next decade. Paper presented at AGHE, St. Petersburg, Florida, March 6-9.

Rosebrook, V. & Larkin, E. (2003). Introducing standards and guidelines: A rationale for defining the knowledge, skills and dispositions of intergenerational practice. *Journal of Intergenerational Relationships,* 1(1): 133-144.

Roth, D. (2004). Young adult college students reflect on their interaction with frail elders. *Journal of Intergenerational Relationships,* 2(1): 29-44.

Senior Citizens America, Generations Together, & Flint Community School. (1998). *Training older adults as in-school tutors.* Washington, DC: Senior Citizens America.

Senior Service America & Generations Together. (2002). *Wisdom works: Training to create a new service built upon between senior community service employment projects in cooperation with elementary schools.* St. Paul, MN: The Pentair Foundation.

Texas Tech University. (1994). *Home economics curriculum, intergenerational professions project.* Lubbock, TX: Texas Tech.

Vander Ven, K. (1999). Intergenerational theory: The missing element in today's intergenerational programs. In Kuehne, V. (Ed.), *Intergenerational programs: Understanding what we have created* (pp. 33-50). Binghamton, NY: The Haworth Press.

Ward, C. R., Los Camp, L., & Newman, S. (1996). The effects of participation in an intergenerational program on the behavior of residents with dementia. *Activities, Adaptation and Aging,* 20(4): 61-76.

Ward, C. R., Walson, B., Nicholson, B., & Newman, S. (1996). *Replication manual: Generations located intergenerational day care program.* Columbus, OH: Generations.

Chapter 9

Defining the Relationships Between Civic Engagement and Leadership in Later Life

Tracey T. Manning

At first glance, civic engagement and leadership may seem to be two separate constructs, only slightly related. Obviously, some leaders are civically engaged and civic engagement can involve leadership, but most people would not see close, or essential, ties between the two concepts either in theory or in practice. It is the thesis of this chapter that civic engagement requires leadership, develops leadership, and would be enhanced among the fifty-plus age group with greater attention to the promotion of their leadership skills and confidence. This will happen only if commonly accepted but restrictive assumptions about civic engagement, leadership, and older adult capability can be modified and expanded.

CIVIC ENGAGEMENT: THEORY AND RESEARCH

Defining Civic Engagement

Civic engagement has been defined in many ways, ranging from a narrow focus on political activity (e.g., voting) to a wider focus also including neighborhood involvement, participation in community organizations, recycling, and civic activism (Schudson, 1999). Youniss et al. (2002, p. 126) summarize their discussion of civic engagement:

Perhaps the fairest conclusion is that there is not a definite demarcation between the political and civil realms. Rather there is a continuum between formal political acts such as voting, political actions such as protesting for a moral cause, and performing a service such as working in a rural literacy campaign.

The Center for Information and Research on Civic Learning and Engagement (CIRCLE) (2003) comprehensive indicators of civic engagement illustrate the possible range from acts of political participation (i.e., voting in national elections, joining a political party, being a candidate for local office) to forms of civic activism (e.g., writing letters to a newspaper about social or political concerns, collecting signatures for a petition, collecting money for a social cause, boycotting products/services because of social concerns).

Civic Engagement Skills

The breadth of possible ways to participate in society leads directly to the question of how and how well citizens are prepared for civic participation. As Della Carpini (2000) notes, citizens require motivation, opportunity, and certain abilities (including leadership skills) to successfully participate in society. To be civically engaged demands knowledge, civic values, and "skills to direct social change in ways that further their vision of a better society" (Boggs, 1991, p. 51). Citizens may need knowledge and in-depth understanding of a particular social/community issue or of how a political process works.

To be involved citizens, individuals also need values that support civic engagement, or as Pratte (1988) describes it, civic virtue, meaning "a civic disposition, a willingness to act in behalf of the public good while being attentive to and considerate of the feelings, needs and attitudes of others" (p. 17). The skills of civic engagement include both interpersonal skills and task-oriented skills that help individuals organize to achieve their goals (Boggs, 1991). In addition, in effective groups, all or most members participate actively to make progress toward the goal (Pearce and Sims, 2002). This avoids the question of whether civic engagement involves followership or leadership; it involves both, though not at the same time.

Effectiveness in a civic group encompasses communication skills such as self-disclosure, listening, assertiveness, and conflict resolution, as well as skills to envision a better situation/world, build group cohesion, motivate others, and strategize toward goals (Johnson & Johnson, 1994; Kirlin, 2003b).

LEADERSHIP THEORY AND RESEARCH

Defining Leadership

Though leadership has been defined in many ways by scholars, there are some common elements to the definitions. Leadership typically involves motivation (rather than coercion) of an individual or group to accomplish a group goal (Hughes, Ginnett, & Curphy, 2002). According to this comprehensive definition, group leadership can occur without a formal leadership position. Also, since group members allow leadership to guide and motivate them, in a sense they are reciprocally involved in the influence process (Rost, 1991). Among the many theoretical perspectives on leadership, those which have generated research most relevant to civic engagement are probably task-relationship/situational leadership, transformational leadership (and other similar empowering leadership models), and leadership self-efficacy.

Task and Relationship Leadership

Early research on leadership attempted to identify leadership traits and explored what leaders (or effective leaders) do differently than others (Yukl, 1994). The recognition that effective leaders behave in task-oriented and relationship-oriented ways was quickly followed by situational leadership models that attempted to identify when to use task and when to use relationship leadership. Task leadership describes the skills and tasks usually associated with leadership and socioemotional or relational leadership, those leadership behaviors that foster collaboration and cohesion and reduce conflict in groups (Fertman & van Linden, 1999). Situational leadership research has demonstrated that effective leaders have both sets of skills, employing them based on what the group needs at the time (Hersey & Blanchard, 1993). In the 1980s and 1990s, as global and technological pressures challenged organizations to innovate, researchers explored models of leadership that fostered change (Kouzes & Posner, 2002).

Transformational Leadership

Transformational leadership describes a potent form of leadership that results in empowering group members to transform organizations and societies. Transformational leaders characteristically nurture personal and group improvement, share inspiring visions of the future, and foster commitment and motivation toward important goals (e.g., Bass, 1985). Described as a mutually beneficial relationship style by James MacGregor Burns (1978), transformational leadership creates an upward spiral of enthusiasm, motivation, and accomplishment. It has a transforming effect on both the leader and the led by raising the level of human conduct and aspirations.

As Burns (1978) described it, transformational leadership is a thoroughly moral endeavor, in which a leader raises the hopes, expectations, capabilities, and moral development of those influenced, who then reciprocally influence the original leader. Though some modern scholars (e.g., Bernard Bass, 1985) would include antisocial leaders, such as Hitler, as transformational leaders, most claim a prosocial orientation is essential to being transformational (e.g., Kouzes & Posner, 2002; Nanus & Dobbs, 1999).

Other theories also make the social responsibility aspect of leadership paramount; for instance, the social change model of leadership and the servant-leader model (Greenleaf, 1977) emphasize the leader's empowering influence on individuals and organizations.

Leadership Self-Efficacy

However, undergirding leadership effectiveness is a sense of leadership efficacy, the confidence that one can help a group to accomplish a goal. Without that confidence, people are not likely to take initiative to make a difference in a group. A relatively new field of leadership research, that of leadership self-efficacy, explores the causes, correlates, and calculates consequences of leadership self-confidence (Hoyt, 2002).

Leadership self-efficacy, drawn from Albert Bandura's work on domain-specific self-efficacy (1977a,b), is defined as "one's self-perceived capability to perform the cognitive and behavioral functions necessary to . . . successfully lead a group" to a goal. Leadership self-efficacy, like other specific self-efficacies, influences much about leadership and group performance (McCormick, 2001). For instance, those with high leadership self-efficacy are more likely to be seen as leaders (Paglis & Green, 2002) and are more motivated to exercise leadership in a group (Chan, 2000). High leadership self-efficacy strengthens belief in the group's potential to achieve, promotes higher group accomplishment, and fosters perseverance toward goals (Depp, 1993; Dickerson & Taylor, 2000). These results apply beyond the business world to community organizations as well. Ordinary citizens with high leadership self-efficacy had greater community participation, and were more likely to be officials and board members, than citizens with lower leadership self-efficacy (Depp, 1993).

The impact of leadership self-efficacy is especially powerful for nontraditional leaders, including women, minority group members, and volunteer leaders; leadership self-efficacy bolsters the leader when his or her ability is questioned and leads to higher group performance (Hoyt, 2002). It seems likely that, affected by stereotypes about older people and about leadership as positional, many of the fifty-plus population would have relatively low leadership self-efficacy, with an inhibiting effect on their leadership initiative.

THE RELATIONSHIP OF LEADERSHIP TO CIVIC ENGAGEMENT

Defined by Civic Engagement Scholars

As mentioned earlier, civic engagement both requires and develops leadership, specifically task/relationship leadership, transformational leadership, and leadership self-efficacy. Civic engagement is often defined or described in ways that suggest/assume leadership behavior. For example, working together informally with someone or some group to solve a community problem, feeling that it is possible to make a difference in the community, or believing in a responsibility to get involved describes both leadership behavior and leadership self-efficacy (Keeter, Zukin, Andolina, & Jenkins, 2002). Specific civic actions like advocacy, mentoring, advising, and community organizing can also be described under the broad definition of leadership (Morone & Kilbreth, 2003).

Defined by Leadership Scholars

Leadership scholars have also made connections between leadership and behavior and how they benefit the community. However, some leadership scholars have attempted to reconcile the perceived distinction between civic engagement and leadership by creating a special category of civic leaders, variously called "citizen leaders" (Couto, 1991), "non-positional leaders" (Astin & Leland, 1991), or "collaborative leaders" (Chrislip & Larson, 1994). Couto's (1991) concept of citizen leadership is complementary to or, sometimes, antagonistic to established political leadership, using civic activism to generate change before politicians or community positional leaders are ready to. Astin & Leland (1991), examining three generations of women instrumental in the women's movement, credited both positional leaders and thought/informal leaders with these social change achievements. Looking at successful community change, Chrislip & Larson (1994, p. 129) credit the collaborative leaders who "usually have no formal power or authority. They exercise leadership in what is perhaps the most difficult context—when all are peers."

Civic engagement and leadership have tremendous commonality without needing to invoke the concept of citizen leaders or collaborative leaders. Mainstream transformational leadership scholars describe the goal of leadership as moving organizations toward the greater good, for the organization, for its constituents, and for society (e.g., Komives, Lucas, & McMahon, 1998; Nanus & Dobbs, 1999). "Leaders are individuals (both adults and adolescents) who think for themselves, communicate their thoughts and feelings to others, and help others understand and act on their own beliefs. They influence others in an ethical and socially responsible way" (Fertman & van Linden, 1999, p.11).

The Relationship of Civic Engagement and Leadership in Youth

Youth programs and research have more thoroughly integrated leadership and civic engagement development than those programs designed for adults.

Programs Relating Leadership and Civic Engagement in Youth

Youth civic engagement programs, whether offered through schools or by national/community organizations, aim to foster civic knowledge, values, and skills (CIRCLE, 2002) and less often intentionally develop the leadership skills requisite for the full range of civic activities (cf. Gibson, 2001). Many such programs do foster proactive leadership along with civic knowledge and community service, though they often miss the opportunity to permit youths to have significant leadership roles in their own projects (Des Marais, Yang, & Farzanehkia, 2000). "We have found that service learning is the most powerful approach in youth leadership development. . . . Through service learning, young people become engaged leaders taking responsibility for solving complex problems and meeting the tangible needs of a defined community" (Des Marais et al., 2000, p. 679). The YELL (Youth Engaged in Leadership and Learning) Program in Redwood City, California, sponsored by the John W. Gardner Center directly connects leadership and civic engagement, recognizing that youths who help to build civic knowledge, leadership, and advocacy skills will be more active in their communities (John W. Gardner Center for Youth, 2003).

High school leadership programs, whether offered through the school or by community organizations such as scouting, 4-H, or the Red Cross, often actively integrate social concern into their curricula or programs, e.g., having students identify, design, and conduct social change projects (Checkoway et al., 2003; Boyd, 2000). A Ford Foundation research report (Mohamed & Wheeler, 2001) asserts that youth leadership programs foster the capacity of communities to address issues and strengthen their futures.

College and university programs often call themselves "leadership" and integrate "civic engagement" into mission statements and programs. For instance, most leadership programs have a heavy emphasis on community service (W. K. Kellogg Foundation, 2002). Some programs/offices even recognize the intimate connection of leadership and civic engagement in their names, e.g., the Office of Leadership and Service Learning at the University of North Carolina at Greensboro.

Research Relating Leadership
and Civic Engagement in Youth

Studies on adolescents support the connection of leadership and civic engagement in youths. As a result of the YELL program mentioned previously, students living in a high-poverty area

increased their ability to manage their time, speak in public, present information, facilitate meetings, work in groups, resolve conflicts and think critically. They also developed greater self-confidence and community awareness as well as a sense of civic responsibility and a stronger belief in their ability to make needed changes in their community. (John W. Gardner Center for Youth and their Communities, 2003, p. 2)

Similarly, students with more service learning experience reported greater increases in self-efficacy and tolerance for diversity, along with greater importance given to community and personal service (Waldstein & Reiher, 2001). Another study found those postservice gains plus significantly stronger intentions to become a community leader (Giles & Eyler, 1994).

Yates and Youniss's (1996) review of community service research found gains in social responsibility, openness to others, and confidence in their ability to contribute to society among youths who participated in community service. Outcomes described in a more recent review of grades K-12 service learning projects by the Kellogg Foundation specifically included leadership development (W. K. Kellogg Foundation, 2002). Conversely, participation in youth leadership programs is linked to growth in civic responsibility as well as leadership skills (Cress et al., 2001). The link between these studies is that both engagement in service, particularly with opportunity for reflection, and involvement in leadership development programs, strengthen civic interest and civic (or leadership) self-efficacy in young people.

Further evidence of the link between leadership and civic engagement in youths is provided by an ongoing longitudinal study of leadership and social responsibility in 500 diverse high school students (Manning, 2004). Both task/relationship leadership and transformational leadership, along with previous volunteer and extracurricular involvement, related to students' intentions to engage in a wide range of civic and political activities as adults. Although the civic value of contributing to one's *country* was predicted only by previous volunteer experiences, adolescents' belief in the importance of contributing to *society* was predicted by their transformational leadership as well as by volunteer experiences. Apparently, transformational leadership in adolescents predicts a broader social concern, not the more limited, ethnocentric concern.

In summary, for youths, both theory and research link leadership with civic engagement, while programs at the high school and college level concurrently foster both civic engagement and leadership self-efficacy. Since adult civic engagement is predicted by youth involvement (e.g., Kirlin, 2003a; McAdam, 1988), leadership is likely to be linked to civic engagement in adulthood.

How Civic Engagement and Leadership Are Related in Adulthood

Programs

Adult civic education programs have not generally made the same connection as youth programs have between civic engagement and leadership. However, both adult education and extension professionals have engaged in discussion about the need to develop civic engagement and leadership in citizens (e.g., Boggs, 1991; Kelsey, 2002). As Boggs (1991, p. 47) notes,

> the quality of democracy seems to depend upon the degree to which civic education can assist adult citizens in finding meaningful bases for participation in public affairs. . . . It requires skills necessary to function successfully in groups and to contribute effectively to their work.

Kelsey (2002, p. 2) critiques the land-grant university extension program for "failing to remember its roots of building active citizenship through the development of human capital that is empowered and socially engaged." The connection between civic engagement, leadership competence, and leadership self-efficacy is implicit in these adult programs.

Research

Considerable research supports the relationship of leadership to adult civic engagement. People who participated in social movements when they were younger (e.g., Vietnam War protestors, Civil Rights activists, women's movement participants) are later considerably more active and involved in community leadership roles than those in their cohort who were less or not involved in social movements (e.g., Hasso, 2001; Youniss et al., 2002). The most likely explanation is that leadership skills and leadership self-efficacy were developed through those experiences. This perspective is supported by participants in a Palestinian women's movement who attribute their nonstereotypic views on women and their high self-efficacy to participation in the movement (Hasso, 2001).

Similarly, a large body of research indicates that adult civic engagement is predicted by youth involvement in high school extracurricular activities (e.g., Kirlin, 2003a; Youniss et al., 2002). Youniss et al. (2002, p. 132) point to the engagement of those who were involved as adolescents either in social movements or volunteer experiences to conclude that service is "an opportunity for youth to develop their identity within a community context, not as a self-enclosed individual achievement, but rather as a social identification that transcends a given moment in time." They suggest that the reason that adolescent activities seem to have a lifelong impact is that adolescents incorporate their experiences of involvement and effectiveness into a social identity, seeing themselves as both concerned about and able to contribute to the community (Youniss et al., 2002).

Experiences of adult civic engagement also have an impact on adult leadership. Adults involved in community organizations described as activist (e.g., political campaigns, environmental organizations) were higher in "political efficacy," belief in their ability to make a difference, and belief that the system would be responsive to change, than those involved in "nonissue" community organizations (Zimmerman, 1989). Research on older adult volunteerism finds that most are continuing a pattern of community activity begun much earlier in life (e.g., Chambré, 1993; Boggs, Rocco, & Spangler, 1995).

Elected officials, particularly women, have a history of civic engagement which is often seen as the source of their leadership. Female state legislative committee chairs were much more likely than male committee chairs to attribute their leadership skills (and by extension, self-efficacy) to their volunteer and community involvement (Rosenthal, 1998).

Outcomes assessment of Project REACH, which trained community-based lay health educators, indicated that both support from the medical establishment and knowledge gained from the educational program helped them take leadership roles in their communities (Hale et al., 1997). Program directors "were able to identify volunteers from a racially and religiously diverse group of institutions and provide them with enough information and resources that they felt prepared to assume leadership roles in developing health education and illness prevention/management programs in their own communities" (Hale et al., 1997, p. 686). The role of knowledge and encouragement in developing leadership self-efficacy in this program is apparent.

Both programs and research demonstrate the dynamic interaction of leadership and civic engagement, and illustrate the necessity of helping adults continue their development. However, it is even more important to deliberately foster these connections in the fifty-plus population to promote an explosion of social capital to benefit organizations and communities.

Civic Engagement and Leadership in the Fifty-Plus Population

Although in the United States civic participation is higher in older adults than in other generations (Keeter et al., 2002), narrow societal and individual beliefs about leadership and about older adults probably inhibit fuller utilization of civic capacity in the fifty-plus age group (Nunn, 2002). Beyond service to the family, diverse roles for older adults include employment, volunteer work, advocacy, membership on advisory boards, committees, or task forces, and community organizing, among others (Morone & Kilbreth, 2003; Schultz & Galbraith, 1993). Though millions of fifty-plus people currently engage in these endeavors, how much more social capital would be generated by increasing the leadership self-efficacy of both current participants and those who are doing little?

Besides lower self-efficacy, another inhibiting factor on older adult civic engagement is a paucity of meaningful volunteer roles. For instance, in one recent AARP survey (Duka & Nicholson, 2002), 41 percent of age fifty-plus respondents worried about not being productive in retirement years. Relative to that, Morris & Caro (1996) describe the vicious cycle that often occurs when organizations with low expectations of senior adult volunteers offer them relatively noncritical and/or routine tasks, which don't engage the volunteers, leading to lower volunteer motivation, performance, and retention. Descriptions of and research on effective senior volunteer programs shows the impressive contributions that can result from developing civic knowledge, leadership competence, and leadership self-efficacy in over fifties and matching volunteers to substantive volunteer responsibilities (e.g., Schultz & Galbraith, 1993).

Programs Relating Leadership and Civic Engagement
in Fifty-Plus Adults

A number of programs have had as their mission the simultaneous development of civic engagement and leadership in the fifty-plus age group (e.g., Epstein, West, & Riegel, 2000; Schultz & Galbraith, 1993; Thompson & Wilson, 2001; Baker, Leitner, & McAuley, 2001). Among them are the Legacy Leadership Institutes (LLI, see Chapter 5), Leadership Enhancement for the Active Retired (LEAR), the Oklahoma Aging Advocacy Leadership Academy, and the Institute for Senior Action. Some of these are more narrowly focused than others; the two most general seem to be Legacy Leadership Institutes and the LEAR program.

Legacy Leadership Institutes, developed by the University of Maryland Center on Aging, combine lifelong learning with civic engagement and leadership development (Wilson & Simson, 2003). Six variations of Legacy Leadership Institutes are already in operation, each focused on different social/community issues and roles: legislative participation, environmental stewardship, nonprofit management assistance, nonprofit coaching, and humor practices for healthy living. Legacy Leadership Institutes directly address the needs of the fifty-plus population to develop three critical aspects of volunteer leadership effectiveness: task/organizational knowledge, leadership skill development, and leadership self-efficacy. All programs include didactic and experiential classes to provide volunteers with needed content and organizational knowledge, leadership assessment and leadership development workshops, skills development for specific volunteer roles, and closely supervised field placements with regularly scheduled reflection and feedback sessions.

The LEAR program

> was established with the fundamental goal of developing civic efficacy; that is, it was assumed that the primary barrier to individual participation and leadership in community affairs was a lack of confidence in one's ability to make a difference in social and political activities. (Schultz & Galbraith, 1993, p. 478)

The LEAR program identified elements of effective community leadership training for older adults, including fostering motivation to get involved in community leadership roles, encouraging awareness of the match between their abilities and community needs, and building competence and confidence through practical experiences like small group exercises, role-playing, and simulations (Schultz & Galbraith, 1993).

Some programs (e.g., the Institute for Senior Action and the Oklahoma Aging Advocacy Leadership Academy) help older adults develop the knowledge and skills needed to be instrumental in political advocacy and policymaking (Baker et al., 2001; Epstein et al., 2000). Participants in these programs, usually already community activists, go through weeks-long training to learning about aging policy issues and social action strategies to influences policy (Baker et al., 2001; Epstein et al., 2000).

Research Relating Leadership and Civic Engagement in Fifty-Plus Adults

Research on civic engagement and leadership in the fifty-plus age group includes outcome assessments of previously mentioned programs as well as studies of civic leaders. Results of both types of studies lead back to the dynamic influence of civic engagement and leadership development.

Research on the impact of leadership development programs for the fifty-plus age group. These studies mostly focus on individual rather than community outcomes, particularly the attitudes and roles taken by program graduates. For instance, after the LEAR program, researchers explored what factors influenced program graduates who then assumed civic leadership roles from those who didn't (Schultz & Galbraith, 1993). Those most likely to take on civic leadership roles after the program were those (mostly women) who had *not* had work leadership roles, previous leadership training, or community leadership positions prior to retirement (i.e., those who might be assumed to be lowest in civic leadership self-efficacy at the start of the program). The program had less impact on the civic leadership of men and women who entered the program with work or community leadership experience (Schultz & Galbraith, 1993). Participants reported that they increased in self-confidence and motivation through the encouragement of speakers and trainers, and gained specific civic skills, such as critical thinking and group skills (Schultz & Galbraith, 1993).

Similarly, participants in three Legacy Leadership Institutes reported significantly increased transformational leadership skills: challenging organizational process (and themselves), envisioning a desired future for the organization, empowering others' leadership, helping groups and individuals with action planning, and positively motivating others. The greatest increases occurred among Legacy Leadership Institute participants not previously in management positions, those who'd been involved in citizens' groups, and those who were less educated. These results are similar to the LEAR program outcomes, in that Legacy Leadership programs had the most positive impact on the leadership competence and self-efficacy of those whose previous experience didn't foster leadership self-efficacy. Those with less education strengthened their leadership skills the most, which could indicate that they gained more from the program or that they recognized leadership competence in themselves that they'd previously underestimated, because of their lower educational achievement.

In contrast to the LEAR outcomes, Legacy Leadership programs had a more significant impact on the leadership development of men who had not held leadership roles prior to retirement. This may be because most women in the LLI programs held preretirement leadership roles.

Another connection was reported between leadership and civic engagement for the Legacy Leaders. Participants' community involvement scale scores (see Chapter 10 for a description of the instrument) were significantly related to incoming measures of group leadership self-efficacy and of field experience self-efficacy. These two self-efficacy measures were each highly reliable and somewhat correlated, though not overlapping. Items on the group leadership self-efficacy scale asked about confidence in specific tasks such as motivating a group, helping a group work out a conflict, aiding a group to envision its future, helping a group devise an effective strategy to reach a goal, etc. The field experience self-efficacy scale asked participants how confident they were about various aspects of their upcoming field placements: accomplishing assigned tasks, building informal alliances, influencing the tasks they were given, and communicating to supervisors. The greater the participants' prior civic engagement, the more confident they felt in both their group leadership skills and in successfully performing in their field placement.

However, community involvement was not significantly correlated with Legacy Leaders' preprogram transformational leadership ratings. This suggests that their previous community experience equipped Legacy Leadership participants with self-efficacy to work well with groups and perform in their field placement, rather than with self-perceived transformational leadership. Transformational leadership competence was apparently gained through training and feedback in the program itself, perhaps as they redefined leadership to include a broader array of skills and roles making up leadership.

Best practices leadership programs. These outcome assessments seem to indicate that effective senior volunteer leadership programs implicitly utilize one or more of Bandura's (1977b) strategies for increasing specific self-efficacy. These include enactive mastery (practicing new leadership skills, using new knowledge), observation learning (watching and learning from leadership experts), social persuasion (encouragement and positive feedback on leadership skill use), and physiological/emotional state (increasing volunteers' comfort level for using leadership skills). Volunteer supervision that increases leadership self-efficacy includes giving specific feedback to the volunteer about her or his effectiveness, along with constructive criticism. Gradually increasing responsibilities after an extended orientation/training will increase volunteers' comfort, leading to attributions of "I can do this."

Research exploring community leadership correlates. Other research explores the factors distinguishing older adults engaged in community leadership from those who are not. For instance, similar to the Legacy Leadership Institute finding, the more adults (from young adults to those over sixty-five) participated in community activities, the greater their perceived leadership competence and political efficacy (Speer, Jackson, & Peterson, 2001). Chetkow-Yanoov (1986) found that older professionals in four fields who continued to take leadership in civic, governmental, or professional organizations in Israel were more likely to be optimistic (including aspects of self-efficacy) and healthy than those similar professionals who didn't continue leading. Those who took leadership roles in new arenas had even greater perceived gains in functioning than those who continued to serve in their professional competence areas. For instance, helping professionals who took on organizational leadership roles and public servants who embarked on social cause leadership reported the highest gains in functioning in their later years (Chetkow-Yanoov, 1986). This research suggests that those who pushed beyond their comfort zones increased both leadership self-efficacy and self-esteem.

Additional support for the impact of confidence on civic activity is suggested by research that older adults who were asked to volunteer did so at significantly higher rates than comparable seniors who were not asked (Independent Sector, 2000). An implicit message of being asked is that the asker has confidence in the older adult's ability to successfully handle the civic responsibility. Research showing greater civic engagement by those with more education (e.g., Burr, Caro, & Moorhead, 2002) probably also refers back to the impact of self-efficacy on participation, in that adults with high academic self-efficacy are more likely to have other self-efficacies.

An intriguing exploration of the civic engagement-leadership connection in older adults involved case studies of civic leaders (Boggs, Rocco, & Spangler, 1995). Initially planning to select only participants whose later-life civic leadership was a departure from their earlier activities, researchers discovered that, for most people, civic activism was not new, but related to and built on the civic values, knowledge, and skills gained through lifelong learning (Boggs, Rocco, & Spangler, 1995). Drawing from life experiences of current, historical, and fictional activist leaders, Boggs et al. (1995) outline a stage model of civic engagement leading to civic leadership. Recognizing that not all persons who are civically engaged go through all stages, they are as follows:

1. *Basic needs*—The individual volunteers as a way to meet his or her own needs (for companionship, intellectual stimulation, curiosity, preserving something valued) and the volunteer setting honors his or her values.
2. *Basic skills*—The person has either volunteered or been asked to serve (as more than a member) and uses skills brought to the situation from previous experience.
3. *Emergent cause*—The individual has identified and become engaged by a worthy cause or project and applies previous knowledge, values, and skills.

4. *Project defined*—This seems to be a crucial stage in civic development, as the person reaches the point of needing more knowledge and skills to be effective in pursuing the cause to a hoped-for end.
5. *Project immersion*—This was another turning point for civic leaders in the making, who felt driven to learn everything about their chosen subject to become more effective in working for the cause.
6. *Becoming an expert*—This stage finds the civic leader intensely committed, almost as if to a full-time job, and seen as a mentor/resource by other volunteers in the field.
7. *Becoming an advocate*—Every opportunity is taken, even to working outside their local area, to promote the cause/project.

In these stages, Boggs et al. (1995) describe a credible developmental sequence through which people can move from early civic involvement to effective civic leadership. The stages also suggest a range of intervention opportunities to increase social capital and aid individual movement along the stages. As if in response, Chetkow-Yanoov (1986, p. 72) urges:

> If leadership is indeed as useful for later years as it appears to be, then training for some kinds of leadership might well begin in youth clubs or within junior-high school curriculum's lessons on citizenship and volunteering. During the middle years, schools for neighbourhood activists should include the rudiments of leadership, and urban-development staff should be alert for potential grassroots leaders. . . . Pre-retirement programmes . . . should include some training in leadership.

CONCLUSIONS AND RECOMMENDATIONS

1. Along with youth programs integrating civic engagement and leadership development, workplaces should offer leadership training programs to all staff (positional and nonpositional leaders); preretirement programs could emphasize the transfer of work skills to community leadership roles. The goal should be to strengthen civic values, leadership skills, and leadership self-efficacy. This should be done not to pressure a prescribed form

of civic engagement for all citizens but rather encourage life style choices and decrease feelings of low self-efficacy.
2. Senior programs and civic organizations need to build on Bandura's (1977a) principles. These include enactive mastery and feedback on leadership competence in senior volunteer training to build leadership self-efficacy, and reap the benefits of pro-activity and persistence in civic engagement.
3. Volunteer and civic organizations need to rethink volunteer roles by matching them to the volunteers' skills and interests, allowing volunteers to help develop their roles, and making roles more substantive. By doing so, they will reap the benefit of increased volunteer commitment to the organization, retention, and performance.
4. Grant and policymakers need to address the gap between available roles and engaging roles for age fifty-plus volunteers by funding nonprofit organizational change efforts along with senior programs focused on leadership and civic engagement.

As Chetkow-Yanoov (1986, p. 73) concludes, "the prospect can be further enhanced if we invest in leadership training programmes as part of preparations for the creative use of leisure time during the post-work years. The pool of potential time, energy, skills and experience—appropriately distributed through voluntary and public community settings—might well be the focus of our efforts in the coming years."

REFERENCES

Astin, H. S. & Leland, C. (1991). *Women of influence, women of vision.* San Francisco, CA: Jossey-Bass Publishers.

Baker, P., Leitner, J., & McAuley, W. J. (2001). Preparing future aging advocates: The Oklahoma Aging Advocacy Leadership Academy. *The Gerontologist, 41,* 394-400.

Bandura, A. (1977a). Self-efficacy: Toward a unifying theory of behavioral change. *Psychological Review, 84*(2), 191-215.

Bandura, A. (1977b). *Social learning theory.* Englewood Cliffs, NJ: Prentice Hall.

Bass, B. M. (1985). *Leadership and performance beyond expectations.* New York: The Free Press.

Boggs, D. L. (1991). Civic education: An adult education imperative. *Adult Education Quarterly, 41*(1), 46-55.

Boggs, D. L., Rocco, T., & Spangler, S. (1995). A framework for understanding older adults' civic behavior. *Educational Gerontology, 91*, 449-465.

Boyd, B. L. (2000). *Youth for community action: Leadership for inner-city youth.* Springfield, VA: ERIC Document Reproduction Service No. ED446199.

Burns, J. M. (1978). *Leadership.* New York: Harper Torchbooks.

Burr, J. A., Caro, F. G., & Moorhead, J. (2002). Productive aging and civic participation. *Journal of Aging Studies, 16*(1), 87-105.

Chambré, S. M. (1993). Volunteerism by elders: Past trends and future prospects. *The Gerontologist, 33*(2), 221-228.

Chan, K. (2000). Toward a theory of individual differences and leadership: Understanding the motivation to lead. Unpublished doctoral dissertation, University of Illinois.

Checkoway, B., Richards-Schuster, K., Abdullah, S., Aragon, M., Facio, E., Figueroa, L., Reddy, E., Welsh, M., & White, A. (2003). Young people as competent citizens. *Community Development Journal, 38*(4), 298-309.

Chetkow-Yanoov, B. (1986). Leadership among the aged: A study of engagement among third-age professionals in Israel. *Ageing and Society, 6*, 55-74.

Chrislip, D. D. & Larson, C. E. (1994). *Collaborative leadership: How citizens and civic leaders can make a difference.* San Francisco, CA: Jossey-Bass Publishers.

CIRCLE. (2002). *The civic mission of schools.* The Carnegie Corporation of New York. College Park, MD: CIRCLE.

Couto, R. A. (1991). *Public leadership education: The role of the citizen leader.* Dayton, OH: The Kettering Foundation.

Cress, C. M., Astin, H. S., Zimmerman-Oster, K., & Burkhardt, J. C. (2001). Developmental outcomes of college students' involvement in leadership activities. *Journal of College Student Development, 41*(1), 15-27.

Della Carpini, M. X. (2000). Gen.com: Youth, civic engagement and the new information environment. *Political Communication, 17*, 341-349.

Depp, M. J. (1993). Leadership self-efficacy and community involvement. Unpublished doctoral dissertation, The Pennsylvania State University.

Des Marais, J., Yang, Y., & Farzanehkia, F. (2000). Service-learning leadership development for youths. *Phi Delta Kappan, 81*(9), 678-686.

Dickerson, A. & Taylor, M. A. (2000). Self-limiting behavior in women: Self-esteem and self-efficacy as predictors. *Group and Organizational Management, 25*(2), 191-210.

Duka, W. & Nicholson, T. (2002). Your life: Retirees rocking old roles. *AARP Bulletin OnLine.* Available online at http://www.aarp.org/bulletin/departments/2002/life/1205_life_1.html.

Epstein, D., West, A. J., & Riegel, D. G. (2000). The Institute for Senior Action: Training senior leaders for advocacy. *Journal of Gerontological Social Work, 33*(4), 91-94.

Fertman, C. I. & van Linden, J. A. (1999). Character education for developing youth leadership. *Education Digest, 65*(4), 11-15.

Gibson, C. (2001, November). *From inspiration to participation: A review of perspectives on youth civic engagement.* New York: Carnegie Corporation.

Giles, D. E. & Eyler, J. (1994). The impact of a college community service laboratory on students' personal, social and cognitive outcomes. *Journal of Adolescence,* 17(4), 327-339.

Greenleaf, R. K. (1977). *Servant leadership.* Mahwah, NJ: Paulist Press.

Hale, W. D., Bennett, R. G., Oslos, N. R., Cochran, C. D., & Burton, J. R. (1997). Project REACH: A program to train community-based lay health educators. *The Gerontologist,* 37(5), 683-687.

Hasso, F. S. (2001). Feminist generations? The long-term impact of social movement involvement on Palestinian women's lives. *American Journal of Sociology,* 107(3), 586-611.

Hersey, P. & Blanchard, K. H. (1993). *Management of organizational behavior* (Sixth edition). Englewood Cliffs, NJ: Prentice Hall.

Hoyt, C. (2002). Women leaders: The role of stereotype activation and leadership self-efficacy. *Leadership Review.* Available online at http://kli.research.claremont mckenna.edu/leadershipreview/2002fall.

Hughes, R. L., Ginnett, R. C., & Curphy, G. J. (2002). *Leadership: Enhancing the lessons of experience* (Fourth edition). New York: McGraw-Hill.

Independent Sector. (2000). *America's senior volunteers: Civic participation is for life.* Washington, DC: Independent Sector.

John W. Gardner Center for Youth and Their Communities. (2003). Redwood YELL project report. Available online at http://gardnercenter.stanford.edu/ support_community/red_yell.html.

Johnson, D. W. & Johnson, F. P. (1994). *Joining together: Group theory and group skills* (Fifth edition). Needham Heights, MA: Allyn & Bacon.

Keeter, S., Zukin, C., Andolina, M., & Jenkins, K. (2002). *The civic and political health of the nation: A generational portrait.* College Park, MD: The Center for Information and Research on Civic Learning and Engagement.

Kelsey, K. D. (2002). What is old is new again: Cooperative extension's role in democracy building through civic engagement. *Journal of Extension,* 40(4), 1-5.

Kirlin, M. (2003a). *The role of adolescent extracurricular activities in adult political engagement.* College Park, MD: Center for Information and Research on Civic Learning and Engagement.

Kirlin, M. (2003b). *The role of civic skills in fostering civic engagement.* College Park, MD: Center for Information and Research on Civic Learning and Engagement.

Komives, S., Lucas, N., & McMahon, T. (1998). *Exploring leadership.* San Francisco, CA: Jossey-Bass Publishers.

Kouzes, J. M. & Posner, B. Z. (2002). *The leadership challenge: How to get extraordinary things done in organization* (Third edition). San Francisco, CA: Jossey-Bass Publishers.

Manning, T. T. (2004). *Relationship of leadership skills, volunteer and extracurricular activities to civic engagement.* College Park, MD: University of Maryland.

McAdam, D. (1988). *Freedom summer.* New York: Oxford University Press.

McCormick, M. J. (2001). Self-efficacy and leadership effectiveness: Applying social cognitive theory to leadership. *Journal of Leadership Studies,* 8(1), 22-33.

Mohamed, I. A. & Wheeler, W. (2001). *Broadening the bounds of youth development: Youth as engaged citizens.* Chevy Chase, MD: Ford Foundation and Innovation Center for Community and Youth Development.

Morone, J. A. & Kilbreth, E. H. (2003). Power to the people? Restoring citizen participation. *Journal of Health Politics, Policy and Law,* 28(2-3), 271-288.

Morris, R. & Caro, F. G. (1996, Winter). Productive retirement: Stimulating greater volunteer efforts to meet national needs. *The Journal of Volunteer Administration,* 2, 5-13.

Nanus, B. & Dobbs, S. M. (1999). *Leaders who make a difference.* San Francisco, CA: Jossey-Bass Publishers.

Nunn, M. (2002). Volunteering as a tool for building social capital. *The Journal of Volunteer Administration,* 20(4), 14-20.

Paglis, L. L. & Green, S. G. (2002). Leadership self-efficacy and managers' motivation for leading change. *Journal of Organizational Behavior,* 23, 215-235.

Pearce, C. L. & Sims, H. P. (2002). Vertical vs. shared leadership as predictors of the effectiveness of change management teams: An examination of aversive, directive, transactional, transformational, and empowering leader behaviors. *Group Dynamics: Theory, Research and Practice,* 6(2), 172-197.

Pratte, R. (1988). *The civic imperative.* New York: Teachers College Press.

Rost, J. (1991). *Leadership for the twenty-first century.* Westport, CT: Greenwood Publishing Group, Inc.

Schudson, M. (1999). *The good citizen: A history of American civil life.* Cambridge, MA: Harvard University Press.

Schultz, C. M. & Galbraith, M. W. (1993). Community leadership education for older adults: An exploratory study. *Educational Gerontology,* 19(6), 473-488.

Speer, P. W., Jackson, C. B., & Peterson, N. A. (2001). The relationship between social cohesion and empowerment: Support and new implications for theory. *Health Education and Behavior,* 28(6), 716-732.

Thompson, E. & Wilson, L. (2001). The potential of older volunteers in long-term care. *Generations,* 25(1), 58-63.

W. K. Kellogg Foundation. (2002, February). *Retrospective evaluation of K-12 service learning projects, 1990- 2000.* Available online at http://www.wkkf.org/Pubs/PhilVol/Pub3762.pdf.

Waldstein, F. A. & Reiher, T. C. (2001). Service-learning and students' civic and personal development. *Journal of Experiential Education,* 24(1), 7-13.

Wilson, L. B. & Simson, S. (2003). Combining lifelong learning with civic engagement: A university-based model. *Gerontology and Geriatrics Education,* 24(1), 47-61.

Yates, M. & Youniss, J. (1996). A developmental perspective on community service in adolescence. *Social Development,* 5(1), 85-111.

Youniss, J., Bales, S., Christmas-Best, V., Diversi, M., McLaughlin, M., & Silbereisen, R. (2002). Youth civic engagement in the twenty-first century. *Journal of Research on Adolescence,* 12(1), 121-148.

Yukl, G. A. (1994). *Leadership in organizations* (Third edition). Englewood Cliffs, NJ: Prentice Hall.

Zimmerman, M. A. (1989). The relationship between political efficacy and citizen participation: Construct validation studies. *Journal of Personality Assessment,* 53(3), 554-566.

PART V:
NATIONAL AND GLOBAL AGENDAS

Chapter 10

Research Issues in Civic Engagement: Outcomes of a National Agenda-Setting Meeting

Laura B. Wilson
David B. Rymph

INTRODUCTION

Each year more Americans participate in some form of intensive national and community service. The Corporation for National and Community Service (CNCS) organizes and supports much of this service activity. In 2004 over 75,000 people joined AmeriCorps, the federal national service program, for part-time and full-time terms of service ranging from a summer to a year. The value and impact of this type of service program is just beginning to be studied and documented.

A small group of institutions interested in encouraging research on service was brought together by the CNCS to sponsor a research forum in Minneapolis, Minnesota, in 2001. The sponsors for the forum included: the Association for Research on Nonprofit Organizations and Voluntary Action (ARNOVA), the Grantmaker Forum on Community and National Service, the Independent Sector, the Points of Light Foundation, and the School of Public and Environmental Affairs at Indiana University. Participation was by invitation and approximately fifty scholars and foundation representatives attended. A range of disciplines and research interests was represented at the meeting, including anthropology, economics, political science, psychology, and sociology. Participants came from both small and large institutions of higher education, research corporations, professional associations, and government agencies.

The four goals of the meeting were as follows:

1. Build on the existing research base on national and community service.
2. Create new networks in national service by bringing researchers and funders together.
3. Define research priorities for the field of national and community service.
4. Develop priorities for infrastructure to support service research.

In developing plans for the forum, organizers recognized that service could be defined broadly with a variety of meanings within different community and organizational contexts. They acknowledged the value of the full spectrum of volunteer and service behaviors. This spectrum includes individuals who host a bake sale for their charities, those who volunteer a year or more of service in exchange for a small stipend, and those who devote their life to public service.

For the purpose of this event, the focus was on structured, sustained, and organized volunteering that involves a consistent, intense commitment over a period of at least nine months. Examples of high-intensity service organizations include AmeriCorps, Senior Corps, Civilian Conservation Corps, National Health Service Corps, and the Jesuit Volunteer Corps. Such service could also include corporate volunteer programs that require long-term, consistent contribution of time and effort and family volunteer programs that engage entire families in ongoing community projects. Finally, the forum was interested in school-based service learning and the role it plays in preparing young people to engage in intensive service later in their lives.

CONFERENCE ORGANIZATION AND METHODS

Participants at the conference received a brief survey before attending the forum. The survey was designed to help clarify the issues and identify additional questions. The survey asked about participants' backgrounds and research interests as well as a definition of "service." Participants were asked for their ideas on what could be done to stimulate more research on service and intensive volunteering. To make the most efficient use of the meeting, the preconference survey results were reviewed, summarized, and results made available as a starting point for specific discussions and work sessions throughout the conference.

The participants also received two documents intended to help fulfill the first goal of the conference, to build on the existing research base: (1) *The State of Service-Related Research: Opportunities to Build a Field* (Grantmaker Forum on Community and National Service, 2000), and (2) *Bibliography of Research on National Service* (Perry, 2001). These documents were produced by James Perry of the Institute for the Study of Government and the Nonprofit Sector at Indiana University. The researchers developed a comprehensive database of 2,559 records regarding research on citizen service completed since 1990. The Grantmaker Forum study concluded that the research to date on service does not offer reliable conclusions about its impact on society or the individual or best practices. Specific conclusions acknowledge the existence of a wide variety of survey, case study, and evaluation reports. Few are based on rigorous scientific studies, perhaps because of the lack of available funding to conduct such studies. The report concluded that there are issues regarding common terminology, lack of infrastructure, lack of interdisciplinary dialogue, and lack of rigorous methodology.

These conclusions provided a framework for the agenda for the conference. To emphasize their importance, the conference facilitator summarized the main findings of the study at the beginning of the forum workday. Key sessions of the day included work sessions on identifying challenges to service research, generating and prioritizing research, determining what kind of an infrastructure would be necessary to foster significant research on service, and determining next steps. Within this context, the next goals of the conference were addressed: identifying research priorities and building infrastructure. The fourth goal, creating new networks, was achieved in several ways. For each major work session within the conference, participants were assigned through random selection to a small group of eight. Throughout the day, groups changed and worked with a different configuration of attendees. Informal opportunities were created through meals and breaks for network development.

Following the review of the Grantmaker Forum study, members were asked to think individually and as a small group about the driving forces and restraining forces in service research. Groups were asked to discuss challenges and opportunities that would affect planning. After reporting the findings, participants changed small groups to engage in the most time-intensive portion of the agenda, identifying research priorities. As a starting point to this task, each group received a copy of the list of research ideas that emerged from the preconference survey completed by attendees. This list was created by combining all ideas suggested by participants without significantly changing or reclassifying any research priorities. Participants were asked to review the list and add any research ideas that might be missing.

Each person then used color-coded dots to vote for the priority research needs in the field. The dots were distributed to match the categories of researchers and funders participating in the conference to determine priority differences for the individual groups. After all individuals identified their priorities, each small group worked toward limiting their findings to five top areas for the group as a whole. Those priorities were written on cards and posted. Each group explained how it had come to its five priorities and what those priorities were. Each group discussed approaches to conducting the research outlined and reported the results of the discussion.

Attendees changed small group configurations again for the last activity—building infrastructure. A list of infrastructure ideas from the preconference survey was provided. Groups were asked to brainstorm additional ideas for creating the infrastructure necessary to support significant service research nationally. The additional ideas were added to the infrastructure list. Groups discussed the priorities for infrastructure that would best serve advancement of a research agenda in service.

The last step of the conference was to ask for individual input. Each attendee received index cards. Individuals were invited to recommend the next steps needed to organize and augment service research. Cards were turned in to conference organizers.

FINDINGS

Challenges and Opportunities

Nine groups of six persons each worked first individually and then as a small group to identify challenges or barriers as well as driving forces and opportunities to moving national service research forward. The groups reported out to the whole conference. In identifying opportunities or driving forces, several major themes emerged. Most of these themes can be categorized under the overarching theme of increased visibility and valuing of national service. The groups found a need to increase public awareness about the work and contributions of national service as well as the underlying community needs to which service was responding. Groups reported that they believed many people are uninformed about the depth and breadth of national service activity undertaken by all ages of volunteers and are unaware of the potential impact of this service on the communities in which they live.

Related to the visibility issue, groups reported that increasing national service research would provide the opportunity to promote service as a problem-solving strategy. The issues of community need and the ability of volunteers to impact those problems were seen as increasing as more research is conducted that demonstrates the exact degree to which volunteers in national service are able to help. Research that gains visibility would provide the potential opportunity to renew the emphasis on U.S. civic engagement. The concept of national service might become institutionalized and a common, if not expected, citizen experience. Enhanced citizenship and problem-solving capacity facilitated through national service were seen as an opportunity to increase public policy related to citizenship and service. Enhanced policy could increase or create global and faith-based agendas on service.

A second primary area of discussion was the ability to further develop civic engagement and service as a discipline. As national service research grows and awareness about service increases, an opportunity to create a body of knowledge and build a theoretical framework also grows. This creates the potential for the development of a critical mass of research scholars. These scholars could be aided in their work by skilled volunteers who could provide help with data collection and management.

The challenges and barriers identified by the groups revolved around the early phase of development of the field. Because past research had been done in a variety of disciplines, each with its own concepts, a common language or shared terminology was needed to interpret some findings. There was a lack of an integrated vision with few interdisciplinary links regarding national service. According to conference participants this type of research is generally undervalued and not widely supported as an area of significance in academia. Without such support it will be difficult to attract qualified and committed researchers to enhance the field.

Another challenge to research on service comes from the varying assumptions held by scholars, policymakers, and practitioners. The ideas of what service is and what it is capable of accomplishing vary widely. For some it is a tool for change, for some its import revolves around individual benefits, and for others it is a form of civic capital. These varying assumptions complicate determining how success is defined when studying national service. The problems in definition are compounded by difficulties in assessing impact in some service sectors. More research and evaluation work is needed to assess impact.

Priorities for National Service Research

Conference participants received an integrated copy of all responses to the preconference survey. Exhibit 10.1 shows the items that were used as a starting point for small group discussions on priorities to which participants could add additional items for consideration. Four additional areas were added during the work session. Individuals were asked to vote within their small groups for the top-five areas of priority. Voting dots were distributed according to three categories: university researchers, foundation representatives, and representatives from other types of organizations. A review of the sixty-nine response items about top priorities revealed eleven areas that received at least six votes from forum participants. These eleven areas are shown in Table 10.1. Results do not include input from forum participants from the Corporation for National and Community Service because the intent was to identify priorities in the research community outside the government.

The top research priority area, the longitudinal study of the effects of service and service learning on stakeholders, received the most votes (twenty-one) in total and the most votes (six) by foundations. Research on the relationship of service to citizenship and civic engagement received the second highest number of votes (twenty) and

EXHIBIT 10.1. Response items to preconference survey question: "In what topics related to service do your interests lie?"

Items included in preconference survey

1. The impact of service on service recipients
2. The impact of service on those who serve
3. The impact of service at the community level
4. How to promote an ethic of service
5. The relationship of service to citizenship and civic engagement
6. Identifying the social problems most amenable to solution through service
7. Finding the most effective structures for operating service programs
8. Identifying the appropriate roles for public and private interests in supporting service opportunities
9. The impact of service learning on students or schools
10. The benefits and costs of service programs
11. The impact of demographic trends and their relationship to service
12. The role of social capital in solving significant social programs
13. Definitional uncertainty in key terms such as *service, civic engagement, social capital,* and others
14. The role of service in aspects of social, psychological, or political theory
15. Nonprofit sector research
16. The relationship of service to leadership development

Other topics suggested by respondents

1. Effective structures for service programs
2. Study the link between American Humanics program, service, and citizenship
3. Policy issues related to the rhetoric of turning to the community to address its human needs through volunteer service within funding support or analysis of necessary infrastructure support
4. Benchmark practices in successful community service initiatives and the thoughtful analysis of the infrastructure that sustains and supports effective effects
5. Outcomes that can be attributed to effective service programs
6. Curriculum issues in developing the next generation of service and volunteer leadership
7. The implications of measuring service by hours and translating hours into dollars and how these equations may actually damage the fragile nature of caring
8. Institutionalization of service learning: how to build this type of hands-on learning into mainstream education, build quality at scale, etc.

(continued)

(continued)

9. What institutional access, incentives, and support are necessary for the creation of inclusive service opportunities?
10. What is the perspective of older adults toward service and volunteering?
11. How can civic engagement—and the specific civic behavior of service—be understood across nations and cultures?
12. Developing and sharing best practices in terms of sustainable, volunteer service
13. Leveraging technology to provide additional opportunities for volunteering and service
14. Creating and preserving a history of volunteerism and service
15. Relationship of service to the survival of our democracy
16. Relationship between volunteerism and family variables
17. What learning strategies are most appropriate and effective for service learning components of service?
18. How can schools be encouraged to develop educational goals and processes for their service components?
19. What are the differences among ethnic and cultural groups in terms of types of service performed and the impact of their service?
20. Determining an appropriate dollar value to place on volunteering and service
21. A series of "stakeholder assessments" of AmeriCorps and university-based service programs
22. Study what service means to the participants, and how it fits in with the other development tasks of their age cohort
23. Establish an Office of Applied Research in Service and Volunteerism
24. How effective are service efforts in solving problems or assisting organizations? Are there models that are more effective than others?
25. A cross-cultural comparison of the concept and performance of community service, including differences among cultural/ethnic groups, recent immigrants, social classes, and religions while controlling for school, community, service activity
26. Study aficionado movements—service not necessarily connected to performing the "common good" but rather out of personal fulfillment or interest
27. Can we learn something from community symphonies for improving service in human and social welfare?
28. Can we better align personal interests with unpaid opportunities so as to create even more incentives to serve?
29. What are the differences in social benefits between service for private gain as opposed to public purpose?

30. Background (personal, family, social, etc.) factors lead some people to see service as a calling.
31. Studies of service from various political positions
32. Studies of organizations (e.g., Catholic Worker; Salvation Army) to learn how they instill an ethos of service and whether and how they have affected the lives of participants
33. Study adults who have devoted their lives to service
34. Study community service programs in workplaces and their links to other service programs
35. A longitudinal study of people, and how people make decisions to volunteer, especially in more sustained ways
36. A longitudinal, qualitative study assessing the impact of the service experience on long-term civic engagement
37. Cross-sectional, qualitative study with a sample of service participants—in different service contexts—assessing their meaning of service and civic engagement
38. How to develop structures and institutions that efficiently and effectively deliver service to our communities
39. How other nations approach service, embrace it, and deliver it
40. Identifying the interests and needs for information and analysis by volunteers and voluntary organizations
41. How volunteer issues are institutionalized in the knowledge generation system of higher education
42. A retrospective study of the difference service makes in the lives of servers including personal choices made by the server
43. Program structure, member experience, and how both relate to member skill development and specific quality outcomes from service
44. Follow-up studies of low-income (precollege) AmeriCorps youths to assess the impact of service on their lives
45. An examination of the impact of AmeriCorps services on selected low-income communities
46. A study of the impact of AmeriCorps service on a sample of recipients
47. Economic consequences to the volunteers of having spent time in service
48. Study linkage between service activity, long-term career development, and community change—with particular attention to how we can leverage service interest among young people by influencing their career choice and long-term career behavior
49. Quasi-experimental, longitudinal study of the effects of service and service learning on all key stakeholders (participants, recipients, community members, etc.)

(continued)

(continued)

Priorities written in by individual groups

1. The political economy of national service
2. Characteristics of effective service programs
3. Improved use of technology to collect, analyze, and share data
4. Study of patterns of service/volunteering at different stages of the life cycle among general population

the highest number (eleven) for university researchers. Representatives from "other" organizations voted each of these two areas as their top choice, giving six votes to each. The third highest area of priority (fourteen) called for research on how civic engagement and the specific civic behavior of service can be understood across the nations and cultures. University representatives voted for forty-five of the sixty-nine areas, representatives from other organizations for thirty areas, and foundations for fourteen areas.

Research Priorities Explored In-Depth

The first round of voting was by individuals in small groups. In the second round, the small groups were asked to: (1) review and discuss the top priorities voted on by individual forum participants, and (2) reach a consensus within each small group on the top-five priority areas. After analysis by the forum facilitators, eight categories of research priorities emerged. The order of presentation corresponds roughly to the order of priorities displayed in Table 10.1.

1. *Rigorous research design and a data set.* The need for rigorous research designs that include both experimental and quasi-experimental designs as well as longitudinal studies is critical. Studies should be large-scale, comparative, grounded in past research and theory, and look to stakeholders for responses. A major data set with multiple components should be created that would include longitudinal research on service and service learning impacts on stakeholders, the institutionalization of service learning in mainstream education, on civic engagement and service, and on cultural and demographic shifts. The overriding need is to build a body of evidence.

2. *Relationship of service to citizenship and civic engagement.* Longitudinal quantitative and qualitative research is needed to assess the impact of the service experience on long-term civic engagement. How do social capital, civic engagement, citizenship, and service relate over time? What is the link between service activity, long-term career, and community change?

3. *Understanding service from a cultural, demographic, and global perspective.* A priority is to create a national and a global picture of national service that provides a cultural context in both national and international settings. This includes: comparative studies, studies that take into account demographics, diversity, international policy issues, and how civic engagement and the specific behavior of service can be understood across nations and cultures.

4. *Impact of service.* Research should seek to understand how national service affects institutions, communities, the volunteers, and the recipients directly involved with service.

5. *Terminology.* Interdisciplinary definitions of service concepts should be created to build a common language for discussion including definitions of service, civic engagement, and social capital.

6. *Effective program structures and design.* Research is needed to help develop structures and institutions that effectively deliver services to communities and recipients including: the development, definition, and identification of best practices for sustainable volunteer service; identification of models that are more effective for specific areas; and analyses of how infrastructure sustains and supports effective efforts; and studies of organizations' effectiveness, structures, philosophy, and outcomes.

7. *Curriculum.* Graduate training programs should build curricula on volunteerism and management of service initiatives to enhance institutional sustainability, encourage effective pedagogical practice, and develop future generations of leaders.

8. *Motivation and meaning.* Little is known about the motivations of service participants and the meaning that service holds for them. Researchers should seek to understand the effects of service on individual learning outcomes and the impact of service on developmental tasks.

TABLE 10.1. Top research priorities according to voting for forum participants.

		Number of votes			
Rank	Research priorities	University (N = 27)	Foundation (N = 5)	Other (N = 13)	Total (N = 45)
1	Quasi-experimental, longitudinal study of the effects of service and service learning on key stakeholders	10	5	6	21
2	The relationship of service to citizenship and civic engagement	11	3	6	20
3	How civic engagement and the specific civic behavior of service can be understood across nations and cultures	10	1	3	14
4	Impact of service at the community level	7	2	2	11
5	Differences among ethnic and cultural groups in terms of types of service	7	1	1	9
6	Longitudinal, qualitative study assessing the impact of the service	4	2	3	9
7	Impact of service on those who serve	6	1	1	8
8	Impact of service on service recipients	4	1	2	7
9	Cross-cultural comparison of the concept and performance of community service among cultural groups, recent immigrants, social classes, and religions	6	0	0	6
10	Definitional uncertainty in key terms such as service and civic engagement	3	1	2	6
11	Effective structures for service programs	3	0	3	6

INFRASTRUCTURE TO SUPPORT SERVICE RESEARCH

With research priorities established at the individual, small group, and large group levels, conference participants turned to questions about infrastructure. Participants were asked to identify (1) the infrastructure that would be needed to move forward on the various research priorities, and (2) what would be required to take advantage of opportunities or to overcome barriers and challenges to research. The forum participants identify six areas of needed infrastructure support:

1. *Annual conferences.* The availability of a specific forum for discussing national service research on an annual or biannual basis was considered. Although a specific conference could be convened, the general group consensus is to attach the meeting to another related meeting in order to achieve maximum effectiveness. A regular conference would provide the opportunity to network, build relationships to create new research, and build synergy.

2. *Online community of practice.* Easy access to and centralization of information is the goal of this infrastructure component, which might build upon other national service Web sites. It would provide a central repository for bibliographies, annotated citations, reviews, online working papers to build the state of knowledge and information, a free LISTSERV mailing list to update information or share ideas, and a newsletter.

3. *National office of applied research.* Conference participants strongly endorse this idea. Such an office could incorporate and become responsible for all other elements of the necessary infrastructure. The office could partner with a university or independent association and provide visibility and legitimacy to service research, and develop a fellowship program or dissertation fund that the national office administers. The office could also pose new questions, generate research funds, create a call for proposals, and help build standards by monitoring quality, consistency, and synthesis.

4. *National collaborative data collection.* As noted in the research priorities, forum participants believe that a national data set could play an important part in moving service research forward. A data set built on existing work such as the Corporation

for National Service longitudinal study could support consistent methodologies, develop a taxonomy for research on service, define terminology, and bridge the discipline-specific work currently being undertaken. With a data set available, funds for dissertations, scholarships, and fellowships might be obtained for work on the data.

5. *Committees.* An adjunct or alternative to a conference on national service research would be committees related to the topic of national service in other organizations, e.g., ARNOVA. Communities could encourage deepening of national service issues and research in specific disciplines or areas of interdisciplinary inquiry.

6. *Using existing professional infrastructure.* Several of the ideas for infrastructure could become subsets of existing activity including attachment to another organization's Web site, creating a section in an existing journal, or creating a pre- or post-conference or subcommittee within another professional organization.

THE NEXT STEPS

Toward the close of the conference day, the facilitator asked participants to write down on index cards their ideas about appropriate next steps. These cards were collected and subjected to pattern analysis to identify the themes that might guide actions to promote the mission of the conference in the future.

The topic that generated the most interest, as expressed in the number of ideas submitted, focused on the need for further planning and coordination to support effective action. Strong support was expressed for reporting the findings and conclusions of the conference, soliciting and organizing reactions to the report, and establishing a planning group to advance the ideas. Some participants advocated forming the planning group from stakeholders in the national service research community. Some suggested that members of the planning group should include researchers, funders, practitioners, journal editors, association heads, university administrators, and selected members of this conference. The staff support could be provided by the CNCS.

One suggestion that was voiced throughout the day: "The forum is a beginning, not an end. We should continue to build a research-practice movement." This momentum was one that underlay the call for planning and coordination and a sense that planning, visible coordination, and open communication are critical to future success.

Many participants felt that immediate communication needs could be met by forming an online community of service researchers under the leadership of the CNCS. The community would build on conference participants and include researchers and stakeholders as the core membership.

Among the ideas for next steps was strong support for convening future forums to keep the dialogue going. Some of those present argued for a forum structure that would include research paper presentations or organizing paper sessions on service at national association meetings. Some suggested that interest groups within associations should be organized around service research issues. Building support in established organizations and associations was seen as critical to encourage university departments to view research on service as a worthwhile topic within traditional disciplinary interests and tenure-track concerns. Two ideas for more formal support for service research were (1) forming an association of researchers on service, and (2) creating a national office on service research that would fund independent research.

Funding was a common "next-step" concern. Several participants suggested that the CNCS broaden the types of research it supports by issuing competitive requests for proposals (RFPs) from independent researchers. The RFPs should seek to fund research in a broad set of areas with its agenda growing out of this conference and its follow-up activities. In addition to federal funds, participants suggested convening a meeting of other nonfederal funders to determine priorities in collaboration with representatives of the service research field. Many conference participants wanted to see the CNCS become more inclusive and collaborative in setting a research agenda, selecting who does that research, and sharing the information gathered by the research.

Finally, some participants offered specific suggestions for research including adding modules to the existing longitudinal studies, doing a longitudinal study with the household as the unit of analysis, building a national data set, and working to develop a common language for service research that would shape discourse across disciplines and types of service.

CONCLUSION

Fifty scholars, foundation representatives, and others met in a daylong conference to discuss the current and future state of research on national and community service. When asked to identify the barriers and challenges to research, they listed: low public awareness of service, the need to promote service as a problem-solving strategy, the lack of a common set of definitions, few interdisciplinary linkages, and varying assumptions about the nature of service.

Two research areas were identified by both university-based researchers and foundation representatives as being most critical:

1. Quasi-experimental, longitudinal studies of the effects of service and service learning on key stakeholders
2. Relationship of service to citizenship and civic engagement

In discussing research priorities, the forum participants identified several issues that researchers should consider when undertaking work on national service including: the rigor of research design; the need for accessible data sets on service programs and members; relationship of service to civic engagement; cross-cultural variables; distinctions between micro- and macro-levels of impact; terminology; effective program design; curriculum development in volunteer management and service; and motivation and meaning of service to participants.

Forum participants expressed a strong belief in the need to build an infrastructure to support research on service, continuing to hold annual conferences, creating an online community, establishing a national office of applied research, building publicly available data sets on service, forming committees or interest groups on service in professional associations, finding ways to support dissertation research on service, and taking advantage of existing infrastructure supports in professional associations.

As a final task in the forum, participants submitted written suggestions about next steps. An analysis of these suggestions identified the following emergent tasks: develop further planning and coordination activities, find ongoing ways for participants and others to communicate about their research interests, hold future forums on research, and seek ways to make funding more available to a wider array of scholars.

In summary, the participants in the forum want to continue talking and working with one another. They want to build institutional support for a more inclusive and open dialogue on service research. They want to be part of a larger movement that builds theory, accumulates a knowledge base on the impact of service on participants and communities, and applies that knowledge to improve the quality of intensive service programs.

REFERENCES

Grantmaker Forum on Community and National Service. (2000). *The State of Service-Related Research: Opportunities to Build a Field.* Berkeley, CA: Author.

Perry, James. (2001). *Bibliography of Research on National Service.* Indianapolis: School of Public and Environmental Affairs, Indiana University–Purdue University.

In summary, the participants in the forum want to continue talking and working with one another. They want to build institutional support for a more inclusive and open dialogue on service research. They want to be part of a larger movement that builds theory, accumulates a knowledge base on the impact of service on participants and communities, and applies that knowledge to improve the quality of intensive service programs.

REFERENCES

[illegible] for [illegible] Community and National Service ([illegible]). *The State of Service-Related Research: Opportunities to Build a Field*. Berkeley, CA: Author.

[illegible]

Chapter 11

Issues in Elder Service and Volunteerism Worldwide: Toward a Research Agenda

Jim Hinterlong
Amanda Moore McBride
Fengyan Tang
Kwofie Danso

INTRODUCTION

This chapter focuses upon individuals aged fifty and older. Although no single chronological age is universally accepted as an indication of having reached later life, under nearly any threshold the proportion of adults considered "old" is reaching historic levels around the globe and is growing at a rate unprecedented in the history of humankind (Cohen, 2003; Kinsella & Velkoff, 2001). Within the next quarter-century, projections indicate that 14 percent of the world population will be over age sixty, and the majority of these older individuals will reside outside the developed world (United Nations Development Programme, 1999).

Nations in Asia and South America will see the proportion of older adults within their populations double or even triple by 2030. These elders will be less educated, less financially secure, and less healthy than their counterparts in more developed areas (UNDP, 1999). Population aging will likely generate enormous strain on emerging economies, and thus may delay or even prevent the establishment of retirement as a normative process in later life. This is especially true within

We gratefully acknowledge the Ford Foundation for its support of the Center for Social Development's Global Service Institute and this research.

countries without national pension schemes. This demographic shift portends significant social, economic, and political change in both developed and underdeveloped nations (Polivka, 2001, 2002).

Previously dominant views of how we should and do grow old are changing, promoting a more proactive and positive view for the potential impact of these changes. These views are giving way to new gerontological perspectives that highlight the importance of continued participation in life activities into older adulthood (e.g., Rowe & Kahn, 1998). This emerging perspective on "productive aging" (Butler & Gleason, 1985) or "productive engagement in later life" highlights the actual and potential contributions of older individuals through engagement in paid and unpaid roles that create goods and services (Morrow-Howell, Hinterlong, & Sherraden, 2001).[1] Scholars in this area have shown that—contrary to myths of dependency that dominate views of the elderly—productive engagement is commonplace among individuals aged fifty-five and over (Caro & Bass, 1993; Bass, 1995). Older adults perform significant but often unrecognized work outside of the paid labor market. Many middle-aged adults desire to remain actively engaged in their communities through challenging, meaningful, and productive civic roles as they transition into retirement (Peter D. Hart & Associates, 1999, 2002).

Volunteerism and service are common avenues for productive engagement in civic life (Putnam, 2000; Putnam & Feldstein, 2003). Through civic engagement in later life, the skills of older individuals can be directed toward pressing social issues and civic renewal (Freedman, 1997) and the older adults may be positively affected as well. Older adults are well-represented among the ranks of volunteers in the United States (AARP, 2003; Independent Sector, 2003). Nevertheless, research on the involvement of older individuals in civic life is only now beginning to accrue, and lags behind the study of civic engagement among young and middle-aged adults. Global evidence of the antecedents, prevalence, and outcomes of elder volunteerism and service is even more scarce.

Civic engagement through volunteerism and service can have a place among the lives of older adults worldwide. These activities are potentially meaningful and beneficial to individuals and important mechanisms for promoting social and economic development (United Nations Volunteer Programme, 2001). Even in more developed nations such as the United States, the call for greater volunteerism and service by proponents of productive aging has been criticized as elitist and only applicable to the lives of more privileged individuals (Holstein, 1992; Estes & Mahakian, 2001). A central challenge is to develop ways of understanding, promoting, supporting, and studying programmatic and policy strategies that foster opportunities for civic engagement that are inclusive of elders in all regions of the world. Any such efforts should be based on clear conceptual and operational definitions of what elder volunteerism and service are, and the societal factors that may affect policy and program development.

In this chapter, we discuss two related forms of civic engagement among elders worldwide: volunteerism and civic service. We consider the issues involved in documenting and expanding opportunities for elder volunteerism and service around the world, and situate this discussion in the context of a "productive aging" perspective. We begin by defining civic service, and then reviewing what is known about elder volunteerism and civic service worldwide. We then consider a range of demographic, social, economic, and political factors that may affect the development of elder volunteer and civic service opportunities. We conclude by positing an institutional framework and a corresponding research agenda.

VOLUNTEERISM AND CIVIC SERVICE: DEFINITIONS, STATUS, AND IMPACTS

Defining Volunteerism and Civic Service

Civic engagement is a complex construct, encompassing a range of social and political behaviors, and volunteering is one of those behaviors. Volunteering occurs in the public realm and has public consequences, and it takes many different forms. Differences in the forms of volunteerism can be construed along several continua, distinguished by structure, auspice and organizational host, compulsion or free choice, time commitment, intended beneficiaries or activities, and remuneration or recognition (Cnaan & Amrofell, 1994; Cnaan, Handy, & Wadsworth, 1996). Variations along these dimensions may differentiate mutual aid, occasional volunteering, and civic service (Tang, McBride, & Sherraden, 2003).

Civic service falls at the structured, formal, intensive end of these continua. Civic service can be defined as an "organized period of substantial engagement and contribution to the local, national, or world community, recognized and valued by society, with minimal monetary compensation to the participant" (Sherraden, 2001, p. 2). Examples of civic service programs include the United States Peace Corps and Japanese Overseas Cooperation Volunteers or national service programs in Ghana or Nigeria. Programs that focus exclusively on elder servers and volunteers are less common but growing in number. Although civic service may share key features of volunteer activity, most notably the performance of activities with little or no compensation. Service is distinguished by its quasi-contractual character, which involves a sustained period of commitment and expressed focus on commonweal impacts.[2]

Elder Volunteerism and Civic Service Worldwide

Proceeding from this conceptualization, what is the status of elder volunteerism and civic service worldwide? Very little research documents these phenomena cross-nationally, although there are a number of studies that discuss their prevalence at national levels and some which explore the latent potential for even greater engagement among elders. In this chapter, we summarize studies that have assessed time use and volunteer behavior of older adults in various countries. We then highlight findings from a global assessment of civic service programs and discuss the extent to which elder service forms a unique group within this set of programs.

Time Use Among Older Adults

Gauthier & Smeeding (2003) present findings from an exploration of time-use patterns among individuals aged forty-five and older in nine countries: Austria, Canada, Finland, Germany, Italy, the Netherlands, Sweden, the United Kingdom, and the United States. Using nationally representative survey data from each country collected between 1987 and 1992, the authors conclude that retirement from the formal labor market does significantly increase the availability of free time for many older adults. This time is reallocated to a variety of activities but predominantly to "passive" pursuits, which include leisure activities, watching television, and self-care. In addition, age-cohort comparisons reveal no significant increase in volunteer activities in later life.

Volunteerism Among Older Adults

The Johns Hopkins Comparative Nonprofit Sector Project (CNP) has assessed volunteerism across twenty-four nations (Salamon, Anheier, List, Toepler, Sokolowski, & Associates, 1999; Salamon & Sokolowski, 2001). In addition to the developed countries of Australia, Israel, Japan, and the United States, the surveyed nations were distributed throughout Europe and Latin America. Data were not collected on the age of volunteers or on whether programs had established age-based eligibility requirements for participation. However, this study is helpful in providing a sense of the scope and nature of volunteerism globally.

Developing countries or those with lower per-capita incomes tend to have higher labor market participation rates among older adults. About 50 percent of men aged sixty or older are in the labor market in less developed countries, compared with 21 percent of men in more developed regions (United Nations, 2002b). Higher labor-market participation may restrict elders of less developed countries from active involvement in formal, structured volunteering and service. Volunteering in these countries is often in the form of mutual aid and self-help, characterized by insurance against future poverty and vulnerability. It serves as the "deposit" in a "social security" system; volunteer work can be used in exchange for future help from others (Second World Assembly on Aging, 2002, p. 2). Through investing their voluntary work, older people in developing countries may be "managing their future risk, at the same time, promoting their own development" (Second World Assembly on Aging, 2002, p. 2).

Research on volunteerism in countries around the world tends to utilize a broader definition of volunteering, referring to both formal, organizationally based volunteering and informal assistance to family members, friends, and neighbors. Rates of volunteering are generally inflated. In Table 11.1, we report national level statistics on volunteering among older adults across nine countries, representing the continents of North America (two), Asia (one), Europe (five), and Oceania (one). The paucity of older volunteer statistics from other countries restricts our ability to globally explore volunteerism in later

TABLE 11.1. Volunteering by older adults in nine countries.

Country	Volunteer rates (%)	Volunteering form	Year	Time commitment	Activities[a]	Source
Albania	3 (65 +)	Formal (NGO)	2001	Unknown	Community development, social services, health, education, advocacy, environment, art/culture, etc.	Dervishi (2002)
Australia	17 (65 +)	Formal	1994-95	100-110 hours/year (median)	Community development, religious-based, recreation/ sports, education, youth development	Australian Bureau of Statistics (2002)
Bosnia and Herzegovina	1 (55-64)	Formal (NGO)	2000	Unspecified[b]	Fundraising, social services, education, advocacy and campaigning, administration, etc.	Kacapor (2002)
Canada	23 (65 +)	Formal	1997	202 hours/year (mean)	Social services, recreation/ sports, religious-based, health	Hall et al. (1998)
Denmark	41 (50-65) 26 (66 +)	Formal	1999	Unknown	Social services, cultural heritage, political work	Norstrand (2003)

Country	Age	Type	Year	Time commitment	Activity	Source
Hungary	21 (61-70 yrs) 11 (71+)	Formal	1993	Unspecified[b]	Community development, education, culture, human services, religious-based, administration, fundraising, political work	Kuti (1997)
Netherlands	40 (55+)	Formal and informal	Unknown	Unknown	Caregiving, local-based, advocacy, intergenerational	Dutch Forum on International Health and Social Policy (2002)
Singapore	21 (60+)	Formal and informal	2000	Unspecified[b]	Human service, fundraising, education, administration, recreation	Applied Research Corporation (2000)
United States	24 (65+)	Formal	2002-2003	88 hours/year (median)	Religious-based, education, social and community services, health	U.S. Bureau of Labor Statistics (2003)

aActivity or organization type may not be specific to older volunteers, but applicable to volunteers of all ages.
bTime commitment for older population is not specified; descriptive statistics may be given for the general population.

life. A comparison of these available data show that volunteerism in these countries varies across volunteering rate, types, and average time commitment and reveals very similar patterns with respect to the domains of volunteer activity.

National surveys in the United States indicate a rapid growth in late-life volunteering rates. The 1989 Current Population Survey showed that about nine percent of older people aged fifty-five and older did volunteer work (Kim & Hong, 1998), whereas 29 percent of people aged fifty-five to sixty-four and 24 percent of elders aged sixty-five and over reported volunteering for organizations during 2002-2003 (U.S. Bureau of Labor Statistics, 2003). The latest survey shows that American elders volunteered with a median of eighty-eight hours in 2002, providing services in religious, educational, social service, and health organizations (U.S. Bureau of Labor Statistics, 2003).

In Canada, the volunteer rate for those aged sixty-five and older was stable over a recent ten-year period from 1987 to 1997 at 22 to 23 percent (Hall et al., 1998). Volunteers devoted an average of 202 hours per year in social service, recreation/sports, religious-based, and health organizations (Hall et al., 1998). In Australia, about 17 percent of older people aged 65 and above volunteered a median of 100 to 110 hours during 1994 to 1995 (Australian Bureau of Statistics, 2002). They were likely to volunteer in social welfare, community, and religious organizations (Australian Bureau of Statistics, 2002). In a national survey of giving and volunteering conducted in Hungary, 21 percent of respondents aged sixty-one to seventy years and 11 percent of those aged seventy-one and older reported volunteer activities in such areas as community development, education, culture, health, administration, politics, and fund-raising (Kuti, 1997). In Singapore, about 21 percent of respondents aged sixty and older reported organizationally based volunteering and/or informal assistance (Applied Research Corporation, 2000). They were likely to be engaged in human services such as befriending and counseling work, fund-raising, and education-related work (Applied Research Corporation, 2000).

Denmark reported a growth in the elder volunteering rate during the 1990s. It was estimated that about 41 percent of people aged fifty to sixty-five years and 26 percent of people aged sixty-six and older were involved in voluntary social work, political work, and cultural and sports activities in 1999 (Norstrand, 2003). Because Denmark is an extended welfare state and the public sector is responsible for social welfare service provision, more than half of older volunteers (15 out of 26 percent) worked in the social service sector (Norstrand, 2003). The Netherlands has a similar level of volunteerism by older adults. More than 40 percent of adults aged fifty-five and over are engaged with some form of volunteer work, but these estimates may be inflated due to the inclusion of mutual aid activities (Dutch Forum on International Health and Social Policy, 2002).

Current elder volunteering in Albania, Bosnia, and Herzegovina is characterized by the involvement and facilitation of nonprofit organizations. In a survey among 360 nongovernmental organizations (NGOs) in Albania, it was estimated that only 3 percent of volunteers in these NGOs were aged sixty-five and older; volunteers of all ages worked on projects in social services, community development, education, employment and qualification, health, environment, as well as other areas (Dervishi, 2002). In a survey of nearly 300 NGOs in Bosnia and Herzegovina, only 1 percent of volunteers identified were between age fifty-five and sixty-four and no information was provided regarding older volunteers aged sixty-five and over (Kacapor, 2002). A large number of volunteers of all ages addressed issues of community development, culture and arts, health and social services, and advocacy activities (Kacapor, 2002). The perception and practice of volunteerism has taken new dimensions in these two countries, which experienced tremendous, war-driven sociopolitical transitions in the 1990s.

Civic Service Worldwide

A recent global assessment study sought to operationalize and identify civic service worldwide (McBride, Benitez, & Sherraden, 2003). Although civic service has existed in practice for centuries, it is an emerging scientific concept (Janowitz, 1991; Menon, McBride, & Sherraden, 2003; Moskos, 1988). There is no agreed upon operational definition. For this study, service programs were defined as those that have a distinct role, where the server is expected to serve for a minimum of one week, full-time, in productive work that addresses important community and national needs.

In this initial assessment, 210 programs were identified across fifty-seven countries; the average service commitment was 7.3 months, full-time. Four of these programs targeted only elders as the volunteers or servers. Forty percent did not establish upper age limits for service eligibility and allowed elders to serve. Nearly all of these programs were explicitly focused on social and economic development goals and activities, e.g., citizenship development, educational and skills training, community development, etc. (McBride, Benitez, & Danso, 2003). They provide a range of incentives and supports to the server including educational credits, language training, stipends for living expenses, and health insurance.

Since the initial global assessment in 2002, we have identified additional elder service programs based outside of the United States (see Exhibit 11.1). Seventeen service programs that target elders as servers were found in eleven countries: Australia (one), Canada (four), France (one), Israel (two), Italy (one), Japan (one), Mongolia (one), Netherlands (one), Scotland (two), Singapore (one), and the United Kingdom (two). The descriptions of these programs were obtained from the organizations' Web sites. Nearly all of these elder service programs are nationally based with few international or transnational examples. Many consider the concept of productive aging to be the impetus and guide for their development and design.

As anticipated, the nature of the service activity and the stated goals of these programs are intended to capture and utilize the experience and skills of the older adults. Older adults in these programs mentor and tutor students, consult with businesses, provide health screenings, assist homebound individuals, and work on environmental projects. There is an intergenerational focus in many cases.

Only one program explicitly stated the expected time commitment; for the others, the commitment is implied. Time commitment may be a distinguishing feature of elder service as compared to youth service with elder service being more flexible (Morrow-Howell & Tang, 2003). Although elder service programs appear to request less intensive commitments, they seem to expect a longer period of engagement. For example, many school tutoring programs require elder servers to commit to working with schoolchildren once a week throughout an entire academic year (Morrow-Howell & Tang, 2003).

EXHIBIT 11.1.
Examples of elder service programs
worldwide by country.

The following descriptions are listed by country, then provide program name, administering agency or body, Web source, and a brief description of the program.

Australia

Retired and Senior Volunteer Program
Volunteering Western Australia
www.volunteer.org.au/volunteers

RSVP aims to provide enriching volunteer opportunities and social networks for mature people. RSVP opportunities are provided by community based, not-for-profit organizations, which establish innovative group projects to utilize volunteers with special skills, experience, commitment, time, and a willingness to learn. RSVP is a service of Volunteering Western Australia and has been operating since 1990. Volunteers assist students with literacy difficulties; serve as mentors for people who have been unemployed and who have business ideas requiring development; aid older immigrants with English literacy and joining in with cultural activities; and provide companionship and cultural exchange to partners of foreign students.

Canada

CESO Volunteer Advisers
Canadian Executive Service Organization
www.ceso-saco.com

CESO is a volunteer-based organization established in 1967. The organization's mission is to promote and assist the economic and social growth and well-being of aboriginal people of Canada and the peoples of the developing nations of emerging market economies of the world. The organization's strategy is to provide consultants that have no private or business interest in the services they deliver to companies and communities worldwide. The role of CESO volunteers is to act as mentors to individuals and organizations in transition. Since its establishment, CESO Volunteer Advisers have completed about 40,000 projects in more than 100 countries using a pool of almost 4,000 volunteers who receive travel and room and board as compensation. Their core values are volunteerism, accountability, transferring skills to people in need, and respect.

(continued)

(continued)

The ABCs of Fraud
Volunteer Center of Toronto
www.volunteertoronto.on.ca/aboutfraud

The ABCs of Fraud program was created in 1996 by the Volunteer Center of Toronto. In 1998, Scotiabank became a primary corporate sponsor. Since the program began, senior volunteers have reached over 68,000 people across Canada. The ABCs of Fraud program is a national consumer fraud education, awareness, and prevention program for seniors. This program uses the skills and talents of volunteer speakers over the age of fifty-five to deliver presentations to groups who want to improve their fraud-fighting knowledge. Subjects include investment and consumer fraud, identity theft, and internet scams. There are currently over 125 volunteer speakers across Canada who deliver the presentations as needed. The program recruits and trains people over the age of fifty-five who like giving presentations and have a commitment to the program.

Senior Peer Volunteer
Seniors Peer Helping Center
www.ssiontoronto.com/agenciesfirms/agenciesfirms.cfm

The Peer Helping Center—staffed by trained senior volunteer helpers who assist other seniors fifty-five years and over—provide individual support, and referrals to appropriate agencies when required; A Time for Me—course providing opportunity for personal growth; Senior Connection—manual for groups, training professionals, senior volunteers.

VIP School Volunteer Program
Volunteer Grandparents
www.volunteergrandparents.ca

The Volunteer Grandparents program promotes volunteerism, and recruits, screens, and supports mature volunteers (over fifty) for intergenerational programs. The program connects volunteers with children and families who do not have accessible grandparents. The VIP School Volunteer Program provides volunteer opportunities at elementary schools.

France

ECTI

ECTI
www.ecti-vsf.org/eng/

ECTI is an independent, nonprofit organization with a mission to contribute to economic, cultural, and social development by providing aid and advice to business firms, and assistance to associations; engages in any initiative aimed at creating jobs or maintaining employment; assists developing countries in setting up a market economy by cooperating with them in the field of economy, science, technology, culture, and humanitarian aid and by striving to create favorable conditions for exchanges and exploiting every opportunity for economic spin-off. ECTI is an association of former managers and executives of companies, government departments, or public services who graduated from scientific, technological, or business schools or universities and have acquired a broad practical experience. Apart from the headquarters in Paris, ECTI has fifty-three regional suboffices throughout France and fifty-four worldwide representations in a number of developing countries. ECTI's representatives are either individual or institutional bodies, who help to promote ECTI's name and services, and act as intermediaries. ECTI's partners include business firms, particularly SMEs, government departments, public services, local authorities, professional bodies, chambers of commerce, public or private institutions, associations and similar bodies, in particular those concerned with job creation, or international organizations such as the U.N., the European Bank for Reconstruction and Development, the European Union, the World Bank, and individual and corporate foundations.

Israel

GAMBLA Program

JDC-ESHEL
www.eshelnet.org.il/en/programs

JDC-ESHEL is a nonprofit organization founded and supported by the Israeli government and the American Jewish Joint Distribution Committee. JDC-ESHEL strives to improve the status of the elderly population in Israel, developing conditions and services to guarantee better quality of life for the elderly, and to improve the image of older people to society as a whole. It has developed many volunteer opportunities for the elderly, including GAMBLA, a program which pairs mature adults with Ethiopian school children. In these special activities the emphasis is on intergenerational contact and enhancing the relationship between youths and the elderly. It is aimed at providing meaningful volunteer jobs for the elderly, and to encourage them to be actively involved in their communities.

(continued)

(continued)

CHAYIL Program
JDC-ESHEL
www.eshelnet.org.il/en/programs

The CHAYIL "Stay Well" program is a grassroots movement of elderly volunteers who press for increasing awareness of healthy lifestyles for the elderly and the development of services to support these lifestyles. It trains independent elderly volunteers to provide health promotion services to their peers. This volunteer program is designed by JDC-ESHEL to help retired people continue to use their education, skills, and experience to contribute in a meaningful way to society. The program is now recognized by all government ministries and nongovernmental organizations. Trained as health promotion activists, volunteers help assess the risk factors, working in HMO clinics to test the balance of other elderly and with local social services to identify accident risks in the home. CHAYIL volunteers also provide screening for hearing and vision. Across the country 500 elderly volunteers conduct up to 10,000 screenings each year, referring thousands for professional treatment—hearing aids, better glasses, cataract surgery—that can compensate for sensory loss and that have a rejuvenating impact on their quality of life.

Italy

Mobility 55
European Commission
www.lunaria.org

Mobility 55 was started in February 2002. It seeks to promote the mobility of European citizens aged fifty-five and older. Mobility 55's objectives include increasing and differentiating training opportunities for those who have retired from the job market. Their personal skills could be a starting point for a newer social commitment, either on a voluntary or professional basis, characterized by a greater awareness of their role in strengthening fundamental European values. Persons over fifty-five can have an international voluntary service experience that applies their skills and knowledge for the common good. Fields include social or cultural work, local development actions, antiracism, reconciliation, education, and environmental protection in countries such as Italy, Austria, Belgium, France, Germany, Spain, and the United Kingdom.

Japan

Senior Overseas Volunteers-JICA
Japan International Cooperation Assistance
www.jica.go.jp/bhutan/senior_volunteers

Japan Overseas Cooperation Volunteers (JICA) began in 1990 to dispatch "senior volunteers" to respond to the growing number and types of requests from developing countries for technical assistance. The objective of the JICA Senior Volunteer Program is to actively support work for nation building and human development in developing countries. The senior volunteers, who are forty to sixty-nine years old, are motivated by the volunteer spirit and possess knowledge and an abundance of experience in a wide range of fields. Their service term ranges between one and two years. Activities are not only aimed at transfer of technology. Through frank communication, they build friendships and intimacy at the grassroots level. Senior volunteers are recruited through a nationwide recruitment campaign in Japan. Assignment of senior volunteers is based on bilateral cooperation between the government of Japan and recipient countries. Volunteer orientation aims to increase awareness of international cooperation, senior volunteerism ideals, history and culture of recipient countries, and other general information. Language training is offered in English, Spanish, Malayan, Indonesian, Thai, Nepalese, French, etc.

Mongolia

Seniors Volunteer Club
Government
www.un-mongolia.mn/~unv

The Seniors Volunteer Club was established in 1999 with the aim of providing health education and psychological support to the elderly population in Mongolia. Training is organized in different activities through the contributions of volunteers who are elderly persons who have chosen to and are able to remain active and productive members of the society. Volunteering activities by elderly persons is a particularly valuable mode of "productive ageing"; their contributions are gifts of life experience, skill, wisdom, and human warmth to other generations.

Netherlands

Netherlands Management Cooperation Programme
NMCP
www.pum.nl/nmcp/index

Netherlands Management Cooperation Programme (NMCP) is an independent organization that assigns senior advisers, many of whom

(continued)

(continued)

are retired or have taken early retirement, to companies and organizations in eighty countries of Africa, Asia, the Middle East, Latin America, and Central and Eastern Europe. These advisers share their knowledge and experience without receiving any financial reward. NMCP is a partnership between employers and the government that was set up in 1978 at the initiative of the Netherlands Christian Federation of Employers and the Federation of Netherlands Industry, which has meanwhile merged. Since March 1997, NMCP has become an independent organization which also provides financial support. In selecting the countries to which it assigns experts, NMCP adheres to the policy of the Netherlands government and the European Union, which together are the main funders of NMCP missions by means of annual grants. Approximately 1,200 volunteer advisers are assigned each year. They are asked to go on missions on the basis of their many years of experience and superior knowledge in a wide variety of fields, such as agriculture, industry, and trade but also in the fields of health care, management, and public-sector services. NMCP determines the length of the mission in consultation with the company in question and the adviser to be assigned. Missions in Europe last for three weeks to two months. In Africa, Asia, the Middle East, and Latin America this is seven weeks, with a maximum of three months. After the mission, many experts continue to assist the companies they have advised from the Netherlands. Only companies that lack financial resources of their own are eligible to call upon the services of an independent external adviser. The company requesting a manager pays the local costs, such as accommodation, cost of living, transportation, and office facilities.

Scotland

Retired and Senior Volunteer Program
Community Service Volunteers
www.csv-rsvpscotland.org.uk

The RSVP (Retired and Senior Volunteer Program) arm of Community Service Volunteers exists to encourage the growing number of those aged fifty plus to volunteer in their local area in Scotland. It taps into the wide range of skills and experience of mature people for the benefit of their local communities. The program is volunteer led and inspired, with local coordinators and organizers recruiting teams of volunteers to address local concerns and community needs. Volunteers help in schools, hospitals, and health centers, transporting patients, befriending housebound people, and carrying out environmental work.

Scottish Senior Alliance for Volunteering in the Environment
Community Senior Volunteers
www.csv-rsvpscotland.org.uk/ssave.htm

Scottish Senior Alliance for Volunteering in the Environment's (SSAVE) mission is to mobilize the energy, expertise, and commitment of older people (fifty and over) to protect and care for the environment for present and future generations. SSAVE is a registered Scottish charity, and already has important international links with similar initiatives in the United States and elsewhere. This program places greater emphasis on involving older people in all forms of community- based volunteering. Working through existing organizations, SSAVE aims to overcome the feeling many older people have that they cannot contribute anything useful to the work of environmental bodies—a reflection of the current emphasis on youth in the media. SSAVE has been established to meet this need through all forms of community- based environmental action. Public understanding and awareness of what constitutes "the environment" is developing and broadening all the time.

Singapore

Retired and Senior Volunteer Program
RSVP Singapore
www.rsvp.org.sg

RSVP provides community-based services to a broad spectrum of society. RSVP believes that older persons are a valuable resource and an asset in our society. The primary mission of the RSVP program is to make senior citizens' lives more meaningful, relevant, productive, and enjoyable through volunteerism. RSVP strives to empower them to become active seniors in community work and encourage them to share their experience, talents, and time for the good of the community. RSVP's approach to volunteerism is different. The program ensures that members volunteer in assignments that best match their talents, skills, and interests. They develop and implement niche programs that maximize the talents, skills, and experience of our members and volunteers. They also dedicate their time to undertake administrative functions with paid staff with many assuming leadership responsibilities. Our support system encourages volunteers to respond creatively and actively to social needs. All of our programs and projects are spearheaded and carried out by members and volunteers with the support of a small secretarial staff.

(continued)

(continued)

United Kingdom

British Executive Services Overseas
BESO
www.beso.org

BESO is a development agency that offers professional expertise to organizations in developing countries and emerging economies worldwide that cannot afford commercial consultants. BESO sends senior volunteers with lengthy experience in professional, financial, technical, and managerial work to developing countries and Eastern Europe. Duration of service varies from two weeks to six months. Travel, accommodations, and living expenses provided. BESO works by matching requests for help from partners and clients with the most qualified adviser, and arranges travel and insurance for the volunteer. Clients provide suitable accommodations and pay in-country costs. BESO volunteers do not fill management roles and clients are asked to provide a counterpart to work alongside them during the assignment. BESO's support comes from the Department for International Development, British business, charitable trusts, and individuals. BESO was founded in 1972 jointly by the Foreign and Commonwealth Office, the then British Overseas Trade Board, the CBI (Confederation of British Industry), and the Institute of Director—whose members still form a strong core on the BESO volunteer register.

The Experience Corps
The Experience Corps
www.experiencecorps.co.uk

The Experience Corps is an independent, nonprofit organization, funded by a grant-in-aid from the British Home Office, set up to encourage all people, aged fifty and over, to offer their skills and experience to benefit others in their local communities. It has an ever-growing range of imaginative and innovative opportunities and projects backed by strong and imaginative marketing. The Experience Corps enlists people who have never been interested in volunteering before or who may have become "lapsed" volunteers. In addition, the organization attracts members of minority ethnic groups.

The Impacts of Volunteerism and Civic Service

What do we know about the impacts of volunteerism and civic service? Mutual aid and occasional volunteerism are more widely studied than civic service, in large measure because they are historical phenomena that are more prevalent and more integrated within daily life. The International Year of the Volunteer 2001 highlights that, while volunteerism overall may be a global phenomenon, scholarship on it is not (IVR, 2002). Because of this international attention, multiple projects have been developed to assess the nature and prevalence of volunteerism in countries around the world.

In regard to civic service, Perry & Thomson (2004) note that there has been significant growth in scholarship over the past twenty years, but this scholarship has almost exclusively focused on youth service in the United States (McBride, Lombe, Tang, Sherraden, & Benitez, 2003; Morrow-Howell & Tang, 2003). The current knowledge base worldwide is thin and claims are tenuous (McBride, Sherraden, Benitez, & Johnson, 2004). We can extrapolate, from volunteerism research with elders and from civic service research conducted in the United States, the possible impacts of volunteerism and service on older adults and those they serve.

The preponderance of impact research focuses on the effects on the volunteers themselves (McBride et al., 2004; Perry & Thomson, 2004; Wilson, 2000). The benefits of volunteering to the older adult are widely noted. Volunteerism is associated with a lower risk of mortality (Musick, Herzog, & House, 1999) and better physical and mental health among older adults (Morrow-Howell, Hinterlong, Tang, & Rozario, 2003; Thoits & Hewitt, 2001). The mechanisms behind these effects are unclear, but several have been suggested including increased self-esteem (Hunter & Linn, 1980-1981), enhanced social status (Thoits & Hewitt, 2001), social connectedness (Freedman, 1996, 1999; Moen, Dempster-McClain, & Williams, 1992), and improved access to social and material resources (Wilson, 2000). Larger-scale efforts to increase volunteerism and service among older adults may be viewed as investments in public health, particularly when these initiatives are organized through policy at national or international levels.

Evidence regarding specific outcomes beyond the individual varies. This variation, in part, is the result of the different purposes toward which service efforts are directed. Sherraden, Sherraden,

& Eberly (1990) note that civic service is utilized differently around the world, e.g., as a tool for promoting peace, improving the common good, promoting state interests, and achieving socially valued ends such as economic development or the remediation of social problems. A growing body of research demonstrates the beneficial effects of civic engagement (broadly defined) on important social development outcomes (i.e., Putnam, 1993; Stolle, 1998; Schuller, 2000). For example, the relationship between civic engagement (or volunteerism and service) and civil society may be bidirectional (Perry & Thomson, 2004; Sherraden et al., 1990).

The evidence supporting the positive impact of volunteerism and service to the welfare of communities and nations has grown so compelling that its role is seen as an essential element of the development work facilitated by the nongovernmental sector (United Nations Volunteer Programme, 2001). Expanding and enhancing opportunities for individuals to engage in volunteerism and service across the life course are now considered among the highest priorities in the global effort to promote civic engagement (United Nations, 2002a).

UNDERSTANDING ELDER VOLUNTEERISM
AND SERVICE CROSS-NATIONALLY

Volunteerism and service are not well-documented cross-nationally or cross-culturally. Scholars are now beginning to study the phenomenon of elder service in the United States and volunteerism and service across the life course worldwide. This work is complicated by a variety of factors, not the least of which is the lack of universal definitions for the concepts of volunteerism and civic service (Dingle, Sokolowski, Saxon-Harrold, Smith, & Leigh, 2001; Tapia, 2003; Sherraden & McBride, 2003). We identify a range of contextual and methodological issues that may affect elder volunteerism and service research worldwide, possibly explaining differences in prevalence of such formal opportunities for civic engagement across countries and mediating knowledge development.

The Relevance of Age

Gerontological inquiry is complicated by the need to recognize and account for the tremendous variability among older individuals.

Aging is both process and experience, present circumstance and history. Individual aging and its collective counterpart, population aging, are influenced greatly by an infinite array of contextual factors. Participation in civic life is shaped by an equally vast set of forces. The study of civic engagement in later life must confront many conceptual and practical barriers.

Perhaps the greatest fundamental challenge to the global exploration of aging-related issues lies in the tremendous diversity among older adults themselves, even those within the same cultural context and age cohort (Schaie, 1998). The phenomenon of individual aging is characterized by a set of universal features that includes changes in physical and cognitive functioning as well as social networks (Hayflick, 1996; Pillemer, Moen, Wethington, & Glasgow, 2000). These age-related changes occur at times and rates unique to each individual (Hayflick, 1996).

Understanding and predicting the effects of population aging are likewise complicated by the fact that this phenomenon is proceeding at different rates around the globe (Kinsella & Velkoff, 2001). The benefits of new medical advances that ensure survival past infancy and into adulthood, as well as those which extend healthy life expectancies, are unequally distributed around the globe. The demographic composition of regions, nations, and even localities greatly affects the extent to which the growing concentration of aging individuals impacts communities and countries. Cultural expectations regarding how age shapes the timing of life transitions and continued participation in civic life also varies considerably across settings.

Despite its importance to discussions of civic engagement within developed nations, age has not been an important focus of comparative research (Fry, 1999). Scholars have devoted some attention to the statuses and roles occupied by older adults in different sociocultural contexts, and have made progress in documenting the utility of a life course perspective in understanding the patterns of activity observed among various subgroups of the elderly cross-nationally (Fry, 1990; Meyer, 1988; Settersten & Hagestad, 1996). The study of productive engagement generally (Jackson, Antonucci, & Gibson, 1993) and volunteerism in particular (Van Willigen, 2000) have utilized the life course perspective to great benefit. To date, few attempts have been made to ascertain the value of this viewpoint to the exploration of late life civic engagement in a cross-cultural or global context. We may discover that population and individual aging are less relevant to patterns of engagement than are cohort and personal history and contemporary contextual factors that promote and inhibit engagement.

Sociodemographic Change

Population aging will generate new costs for many nations. However, this demographic shift is occurring in conjunction with a historic "epidemiologic transition" (Omran, 1971) characterized by a beneficial compression of morbidity that will enable individuals to have longer, healthy life expectancies and fewer years of frailty. Although this suggests the possibility that nations will be able to draw upon a growing pool of talented, healthy older adults, developing nations will also face higher rates of disability among the oldest segments of their populations (Kinsella & Velkoff, 2001). Unevenness in the capabilities of individuals to sustain involvement in productive roles will place strains on public and private systems of care and support. Interestingly, research suggests that older volunteers and servers are particularly effective at addressing the needs of their frail peers (Abraham, Arrington, & Wasserbauer, 1996; Dulka, Yaffe, Goldin, & Rowe, 1999) and those of children and families (Kuehne & Sears, 1993). Civic engagement via volunteerism and service may help to offset the economic and social costs associated with population aging and other demographic changes (Lane, 1998).

Geographic mobility is another important factor contributing to patterns of civic engagement within the United States (Putnam, 2000). Mobility is important to aging individuals and their families (Robert, 2002), but can have negative consequences for community life (Putnam, 2000). In developing nations, a long-established flow of younger adults from rural to urban areas will likely continue and leave older individuals behind in rural areas (Kinsella & Velkoff, 2001). It also counteracts, in part, the trend of population aging to produce greater numbers of multigenerational households that remain very common in developing areas (Kinsella & Velkoff, 2001).

In summary, will movement toward development goals enhance or detract from current and future efforts at fostering engagement? Putnam (2000) asks whether globalization may portend "community life atrophy." It is likely that these countervailing demographic and social changes will lead to new patterns of civic engagement. Even in highly developed nations such as the United States with resources and traditions supporting civic engagement, such activity may exhibit a wax and wane (Rich, 1999) and new patterns do emerge partly in response to such forces (Schudson, 1996).

Variations in Social and Political Forces

Individual and collective civic behaviors are influenced by social norms regarding engagement in public life. Civic engagement encompasses a variety of activities, some of which (i.e., participation in political affairs) may be precluded in certain settings by cultural values or even governmental rule. For example, the value placed on actions that benefit the collective welfare (Funk, 1998) and prosocial attitudes (Penner & Finkelstein, 1998) help determine the likelihood of civic engagement. Cultures and subgroups within populations differ in the emphasis they place on contributions to the common good (Sanchez-Jankowski, 2002). The arrangement of public resources to support service activities is made more challenging in the United States where independent action and self-reliance are emphasized over communitarian principles (Etzioni, 1996). In a similar fashion, the freedom to participate in religious associations is curtailed or nonexistent in some regions of the world. This constrains or eliminates an important social structure for supporting civic engagement (Wuthnow, 1999).

Service and volunteerism are associated with greater political involvement (Wilson, 2000). The extent to which civic engagement of any form is seen as a proxy for active citizenship and concern for the affairs and functioning of the state, the promotion of service may be in concert with or in opposition to the current governing structure. This is particularly true when civic engagement is viewed as a means of nurturing democratic political processes (Almond & Verba, 1963). Mutual aid and volunteerism may still occur, but be conducted generally on an informal basis that escapes direct observation. These actions might serve important ends, e.g., the maintenance of social networks, but may not connect the individual to the public sphere as would publicly supported civic service.

Governmental involvement in the social welfare arena may also influence volunteer and service participation by individuals, although the evidence does not show a significant "crowding out" of private action by public sector welfare expenditures (Salamon & Sokolowski, 2001). As in the United States, public welfare outlays are related to the size and vitality of the nonprofit sector, which makes the greatest use of volunteers. Public investments in other social institutions, such as public education, also have an effect on the availability of service opportunities (Egerton, 2002; Torney-Purta, 2002). Although public schooling may seem disconnected from the involvement of older adults in civic life, research has demonstrated the continuity of engagement patterns over the life course (Moen et al., 1992; Atchley, 1993). Promotion of service and volunteerism among young adults may establish lifelong trajectories of civic engagement.

Over the past thirty years, there has been a significant increase in the number of nations with publicly financed pension plans. Currently, approximately 170 nations have them (SSA, 1999), although they vary significantly with respect to replacement rates (OECD, 1998). The availability of economic support for those who leave the labor market will hasten the institutionalization of retirement in many countries, and in turn make it possible for more older individuals to direct their energies into civic roles. These effects may emerge more slowly in developing nations than they have elsewhere, because in these countries labor force participation rates are higher and more stable, and gender differences in paid employment status are shrinking (Kinsella and Velkoff, 2001).

STUDYING VOLUNTEERISM AND SERVICE AMONG OLDER ADULTS WORLDWIDE

In this chapter, we present a conceptualization and operational examples of volunteerism and civic service, summarizing existing research. We suggest that volunteerism and civic service, specifically, may represent promising approaches to address social and economic issues faced by elders and the communities and nations in which they live, including the impacts of population aging itself. Volunteerism and service produce a range of possible outcomes. The realization of these outcomes may rest on the development of volunteerism and service opportunities worldwide. As we have demonstrated, very little is known definitively about the forms and effects of volunteerism and service among older adults worldwide. The development of effective and efficient opportunities depends on this knowledge. In this concluding section, we offer an institutional perspective, which may support a comparative research agenda on volunteerism and service among older adults.

Institutional Lead

Capturing the productive potential of older adults and directing that resource toward stabilization, renewal, and advance of public life requires access to social resources (Wilson and Musick, 1998) and the creation of social institutions (Freedman, 2001). This has long been recognized by advocates of elder service (i.e., Jusenius, 1986; Morgan, 1986; Sainer, 1976). Institutional change is slow and lags behind the rate at which individual and cohort preferences and behaviors evolve (Riley & Riley, 1994). Perhaps an even greater concern to such efforts is that social policy around the world generally does little to promote, or often serves to inhibit, the productive engagement of older adults (Uhlenberg, 1992). Quasi-governmental groups such as the United Nations are making progress in helping national governments to develop and strengthen statutory and legal frameworks that facilitate volunteerism (United Nations, 2002a).

As noted, strategies for promoting and supporting civic engagement by elders will vary from setting to setting. In some cases, an expansion of existing publicly supported service programs may be warranted. In others, new social structures will need to be created that capture the existing capacity of seniors and anticipate the future demands for service opportunities. Ultimately, opportunities for service are made available to the server by community-based organizations. The availability of opportunities is likely related to the status of the nonprofit sector or civil society in any given country (McBride, Benitez, & Sherraden, 2003). Enhancement of elder service will also require both an expansion of the number and an improvement in the quality of service roles (Morris & Caro, 1996) and new strategies for recruiting older individuals into those positions (Fischer & Schaffer, 1993). In the United States, for example, this latter effort could be incorporated into "life options" counseling (Civic Ventures, 2003), which shows promise as a policy and program innovation. Life options counseling encourages planning for retirement that extends beyond financial considerations to include how an individual will invest a lifetime of experience and time no longer committed to paid employment (Birren, 2001).

Older adults themselves are actively engaged in creating new institutions that enable them to remain engaged in activity with personal meaning and civic implications. Three examples of this "institutional lead" are Experience Corps, an initiative of Civic Ventures, the Retired and Senior Volunteer Program International (RSVPI) based at the University of Maryland Center on Aging, and the Retired and Senior Volunteer Programme in Great Britain (Hoodless, 2003). These initiatives serve to engage the talents of older adults to address needs of local communities. Notably, RSVPI has been involved in creating program-based opportunities for service within thirty nations, making it one of the most successful international senior service programs.

Volunteerism and Service As Institutions: Toward a Comparative Perspective

Volunteerism and civic service are tied explicitly to institutions or formal social structures, which in this context include distinct policies and programs. We offer an institutional perspective for the study of volunteerism and service and identify key dimensions that link the individual to volunteer and service roles (Morrow-Howell et al., 2003). These dimensions include expectations, access, incentives, information, and facilitation. The following section briefly defines these dimensions with an eye toward international comparison.

Expectations include norms and program requirements for role performance that can be formally and informally conveyed through a variety of means, e.g., volunteer position announcements, policy liberties, the family, media, etc. (North, 1990). Access for performance of a given behavior may relate to the sanction or right by a given polity for being a member of society and for behaving in such a way. Access also includes program eligibility criteria, which may be related to the individual's capacity, such as his or her knowledge, health, time, and money (Hinterlong, 2002). Incentives are inducements offered by the sponsoring organization or the individual's motivations, which may be ideological (including personal and spiritual), social, economic, and legal. Information is required so one knows how to act and what one is acting on. This includes how the role has been defined and communicated to the potential servers. Various supports, encompassing administrative oversight, training, and availability of resources, facilitate completion of assigned responsibilities and enhance the likelihood that the server will remain involved in the program.

When these institutional dimensions are paired with the conceptualization of volunteerism and service, a comparative framework is advanced for studying the emergence, forms, and nature of elder volunteerism and service worldwide. The assessment of the continua of volunteerism and these institutional dimensions promotes specification in the study of volunteerism and service. Assessment also encourages a context-specific view on the phenomena, allowing for analyses of different social, economic, and cultural variables, e.g., demographic issues, retirement norms and pension policies, rights, and the status of civil society. An institutional perspective promotes consideration of how policies and programs are structured to support the inclusion of elders with varying capacities. Given the formal nature of service and many volunteer opportunities, the development and refinement of these facilitative structures are critical to civic engagement.

CONCLUSION

Civic engagement through volunteerism and service is a critical issue in the context of population aging as well as productive aging. The expansion of opportunities for volunteerism and service aids in the creation of what the United Nations has termed, societies "for all ages." From a global perspective, public and private efforts to stimulate greater engagement in volunteerism and service will be more challenging in developing areas given the already weak nature of other primary social institutions, i.e., the state, economy, indigenous voluntary sector, and educational system. The expansion of service opportunities via investments in the institutional arrangements must be undertaken concurrently with those aimed at improving the capacity of these other sectors. A related challenge is to ensure that emergent opportunities are designed to promote social inclusion and foster participation in public life among all segments of society, in particular older adults and marginalized communities. Strengthening volunteer and service institutions is a possible means to accomplish important public work, and can act as a bridge between private lives and public concerns. Basic work is still needed in order to document and study the forms and nature of volunteerism and civic service among older adults worldwide and to explore the impacts associated with the forms of productive, civic engagement.

NOTES

1. Productive aging is not a normative perspective that promotes a model by which people should age, but rather calls for greater emphasis on expanding the quality and availability of opportunities for engagement (Hinterlong, Morrow-Howell, & Sherraden 2001).

2. Because of its programmatic nature, our bias is that there may be greater potential for targeted and sustained effects through long-term, intensive civic service institutions. Civic service is designed to provide a formal role for the elder that will positively impact the server and the individuals or communities being served. Service may represent an additional productive role, which utilizes and further enhances the skills and knowledge of elders, provides them with opportunities for meaningful work, and creates flexible and supportive structures that accommodate age-related functional changes or other limitations to engagement.

3. An innovative policy consideration could be the connection between civic service and asset accounts. Most service programs offer stipends or payments for living expenses to long-term servers. Beyond any stipend that may be paid to the server, service hours could be monetized, and based on the number of hours an older adult works, that amount could be deposited into a retirement or pension account. While the older adult is performing important public work, he or she is also accumulating financial support for when his or her health or functional capacity declines.

REFERENCES

AARP. (2003). *Time and money: An in-depth look at 45+ volunteers and donors.* Washington, DC: AARP.

Abraham, I.L., Arrington, D.T., & Wasserbauer, L.I. (1996). Using elderly volunteers to care for the elderly: Opportunities for nursing. *Nursing Economics,* 14(4), 232-239.

Almond, G.A. & Verba, S. (1963). *The civic culture: Political attitudes in five democracies.* Princeton, NJ: Princeton University Press.

Applied Research Corporation. (2000). *National benchmark survey on volunteerism in Singapore 2000.* Singapore: National Volunteer Center.

Atchley, R.C. (1993). Continuity theory and the evolution of activity in later life. In J.R. Kelly (Ed.), *Activity and aging: Staying involved in later life* (pp. 5-17). Newbury Park, CA: Sage Publications, Inc.

Australian Bureau of Statistics. (2002). *Australian Social Trends 1997.* Available online at http://www.abs.gov.au/Ausstats/.

Bass, S.A. (Ed.). (1995). *Older and active: How Americans over 55 are contributing to society.* Chelsea, MI: BookCrafters and Yale University.

Birren, J. (2001). Psychological implications of productive aging. In N. Morrow-Howell, J. Hinterlong, and M. Sherraden (Eds.), *Productive aging: Concepts and challenges* (pp. 102-119). Baltimore, MD: Johns Hopkins University Press.

Butler, R.N. & Gleason, H.P. (Eds.). (1985). *Productive aging: Enhancing vitality in later life.* New York: Springer Publishing Co., Inc.

Caro, F. G. & Bass, S.A. (1993). *Patterns of productive activity among older Americans.* Boston: University of Massachusetts.

Civic Ventures. (2003). *Life options blueprint.* San Francisco, CA: Author.

Cnaan, R.A. & Amrofell, L. (1994). Mapping volunteer activity. *Nonprofit and Voluntary Sector Quarterly,* 23(4), 335-351.

Cnaan, R.A., Handy, F., & Wadsworth, M. (1996). Defining who is a volunteer: Conceptual and empirical considerations. *Nonprofit and Voluntary Sector Quarterly,* 25(3), 364-383.

Cohen, J.E. (2003). Human population: The next half century. *Science,* 302, 1172-1175.

Dervishi, Z. (2002). Volunteering in the Republic of Albania: Reality, ideas, challenges. Available online at http://www.worldvolunteerweb.org/dynamic/info base/pdf/2002/ALB020612_IYV_VolunteeringReference_engl.pdf.

Dingle, A., Sokolowski, W., Saxon-Harrold, S.K.E., Smith, J.D., & Leigh, R. (Eds.). (2001). *Measuring volunteering: A practical toolkit.* Available online at http://www.independentsector.org/programs/research/toolkit/IYVToolkit.PDF.

Dulka, I.M., Yaffe, M.J., Goldin, B., & Rowe, W.S. (1999). The use of senior volunteers in the care of discharged geriatric patients. *Journal of Sociology and Social Welfare,* 26(1), 69-85.

Dutch Forum on International Health and Social Policy. (2002). Factsheet Senior Citizens in the Netherlands. Available online at http://www.ouderenenarbeid .nl/artman/uploads/senior_citizens_nizw.pdf.

Egerton, M. (2002). Higher education and civic engagement. *British Journal of Sociology,* 53(4), 603-620.

Estes, C.L. & Mahakian, J. (2001). A political economy critique of "productive aging." In N. Morrow-Howell, J. Hinterlong, & M. Sherraden (Eds.), *Productive aging: Concepts and challenges* (pp. 197-214). Baltimore: Johns-Hopkins University Press.

Etzioni, A. (1996). *The new golden rule: Community and morality in a democratic society.* New York: Basic Books.

Fischer, L.R. & Schaffer, K.B. (1993). *Older volunteers: A guide to research and practice.* Newbury Park, CA: Sage Publications.

Freedman, M. (1996). The aging opportunity: America's elderly as a civic resource. *The American Prospect,* 29(November-December), 44-52.

Freedman, M. (1997). Toward civic renewal: How senior citizens could save civil society. In K. Brabazon & R. Disch (Eds.), *Intergenerational approaches in aging: Implications for education, policy, and practice* (pp. 243-263). Binghamton, NY: The Haworth Press.

Freedman, M. (1999). *Prime time: How baby boomers will revolutionize retirement and transform America.* New York: Public Affairs.

Freedman, M. (2001). Structural lead: Building the new institutions for an aging America. In N. Morrow-Howell, J. Hinterlong, & M. Sherraden (Eds.), *Productive aging: Concepts and challenges* (pp. 245-260). Baltimore, MD: Johns Hopkins University Press.

Fry, C.L. (1990). The life course in context: Implications of comparative research. In R.L. Rubinstein (Ed.), *Aging and anthropology* (pp. 129-149). Dordreth, the Netherlands: Kluwer Academic Publishers.

Fry, C.L. (1999). Anthropological theories of age and aging. In V. Bengtson & K.W. Schaie (Eds.), *Handbook of theories of aging* (pp. 271-286). New York: Springer.

Funk, C.L. (1998). Practicing what we preach? The influence of societal interest value on civic engagement. *Political Psychology,* 19(3), 601-614.

Gauthier, A.H. & Smeeding, T.M. (2003). Time use at older ages: Cross-national differences. *Research on Aging,* 25(3), 247-268.

Hall, M., Knight, T., Reed, P., Bussiere, P., McRae, D., & Brown, P. (1998). *Caring Canadians, involved Canadians: Highlights from the 1997 National Survey of Giving, Volunteering and Participation.* Ottawa: Minister of Industry.

Hayflick, L. (1996). *How and why we age* (Second edition). New York: Ballantine Books.

Hinterlong, J. (2002). Productive engagement and well-being in later life: A study of activity types, levels, and patterns. *Dissertation Abstracts International,* 63, 3305.

Hinterlong, J., Morrow-Howell, N., & Sherraden, M. (2001). Productive aging: Principles and perspective. In N. Morrow-Howell, J. Hinterlong, & M. Sherraden (Eds.), *Productive aging: Concepts and controversies* (pp. 4-17). Baltimore, MD: Johns Hopkins University Press.

Holstein, M. (1992). Productive aging: A feminist critique. *Journal of Aging and Social Policy,* 4(3/4), 17-33.

Hoodless, E. (2003). Senior volunteers: Solutions waiting to happen. *Service Enquiry,* 1(1), 73-89.

Hunter, K.I. & Linn, M.W. (1980-1981). Psychosocial differences between elderly volunteers and non-volunteers. *International Journal of Aging and Human Development,* 12(3), 205-213.

Independent Sector. (2003). *Experience at work.* Waldorf, MD: Independent Sector.

IVR. (2002). *International year of the volunteer, global evaluation.* London: Institute of Volunteering Research.

Jackson, J.S., Antonucci, T.C., & Gibson, R.C. (1993). Cultural and ethnic contexts of aging productively over the life course: An economic network framework. In S.A. Bass, F.G. Caro, & Y.P. Chen (Eds.), *Achieving a productive aging society* (pp. 249-268). Westport, CT: Auburn House.

Janowitz, M. (1991). *The reconstruction of patriotism: Education for civic consciousness.* Chicago: University of Chicago Press.

Jusenius, C.L. (1986). *Retirement and older Americans' participation in volunteer activities.* Research Report Series, RR-83-01. National Commission for Employment Policy. Washington, DC: United States Government Printing Office.

Kacapor, A.S. (2002). Volunteering in Bosnia and Herzegovina. Available online at http://www.worldvolunteerweb.org/dynamic/infobase/pdf/2003/03_04_15_BIH _volunteerism.pdf.

Kim, S. & Hong, G. (1998). Volunteer participation and time commitment by older Americans. *Family and Consumer Sciences Research Journal, 27*(2), 146-166.

Kinsella, K. & Velkoff, V.A. (2001). *An aging world: 2001.* U.S. Census Bureau, Series P95/01-1. Washington, DC: United States Government Printing Office.

Kuehne, V.S. & Sears, H.A. (1993). Beyond the call of duty: Older volunteers committed to children and families. *Journal of Applied Gerontology, 12*(4), 425-438.

Kuti, E. (1997). *Individual giving and volunteering in Hungary.* Washington, DC: The Aspen Institute.

Lane, R. (1998). International year of older persons. *Social Development Review, 2*(3), 10-17.

McBride, A.M., Benitez, C., & Danso, K. (2003). Civic service worldwide: Social development goals and partnerships. *Social Development Issues, 25*(1/2), 175-188.

McBride, A.M., Benitez, C., & Sherraden, M. (2003). *The forms and nature of civic service: A global assessment.* Research report. St. Louis: Center for Social Development, Washington University.

McBride, A.M., Lombe, M., Tang, F., Sherraden, M., & Benitez, C. (2003). *The knowledge base on civic service: Status and directions,* working paper 03-20. St. Louis: Center for Social Development, Washington University.

McBride, A.M. & Sherraden, M. (2003). Toward a global research agenda on civic service. Editors' introduction. *Nonprofit and Voluntary Sector Quarterly, 33,* 3S-7S.

McBride, A.M., Sherraden, M., Benitez, C., & Johnson, E. (2004). Civic service worldwide: Defining a field, building a knowledge base. *Nonprofit and Voluntary Sector Quarterly, 33,* 85-215.

Menon, N., McBride, A. M., & Sherraden, M. (2003). Understanding service in the context of history and culture. In H. Perold, S. Stroud, & M. Sherraden (Eds.), *Service enquiry: Service in the 21st century (*pp. 149-158). Johannesburg: comPress.

Meyer, J.W. (1988). Levels of analysis: The life course as a cultural construction. In M.W. Riley, B.J. Huber, & B.B. Hess (Eds.), *Social change and the life course* (pp. 49-62). Newbury Park, CA: Sage Publications, Inc.

Moen, P., Dempster-McClain, D., & Williams, R., Jr. (1992). Successful aging: A life-course perspective on women's multiple roles and health. *American Journal of Sociology,* 97(6), 1612-1638.

Morgan, J.N. (1986). Unpaid productive activity over the life course. In Committee on an Aging Society (Ed.), *Productive roles in an older society* (pp. 250-280). Washington, DC: National Academy Press.

Morris, R. & Caro, F.G. (1996). Productive retirement: Stimulating greater volunteer efforts to meet national needs. *Journal of Volunteer Administration,* 14(2), 1-11.

Morrow-Howell, N., Hinterlong, J., Sherraden, M. (2001). *Productive aging: Concepts and Challenges.* Baltimore: Johns Hopkins University Press.

Morrow-Howell, N., Hinterlong, J., Sherraden, M., Tang, F., & Rozario, P. (2003). The effects of volunteering on the well-being of older adults. *Journal of Gerontology: Social Sciences,* 58B(3), S137-S145.

Morrow-Howell, N., Hinterlong, J., Sherraden, M., Tang, F., Thirupathy, P., & Nagchoudhuri, M. (2003). Institutional capacity for elder service. *Social Development Issues,* 25(1/2), 189-204.

Morrow-Howell, N. & Tang, F. (2003). *Elder and youth service in comparative perspective: Nature, activities, and impacts.* Working paper. St. Louis: Center for Social Development, Washington University in St. Louis.

Moskos, C. (1988). *A call to civic service: National service for country and community.* New York: Free Press.

Musick, M.A., Herzog, A.R., & House, J.S. (1999). Volunteering and mortality among older adults: Findings from a national sample. *Journals of Gerontology: Social Sciences,* 54B(3), S173-S180.

Norstrand, J.A. (2003). *Volunteerism amongst older Danes.* Global Action on Aging. Available online at http://www.globalaging.org/elderrights/world/volunteeresm.htm.

North, D.C. (1990). *Institutions, institutional change, and economic performance.* New York: Cambridge University Press.

Omran, A.R. (1971). The epidemiological transition: A theory of the epidemiology of population change. *Milbank Quarterly,* 49, 509-538.

Organization for Economic Co-operation and Development (OECD). (1998). *Maintaining Prosperity in an Ageing Society.* Paris: OECD.

Penner, L.A. & Finkelstein, M.A. (1998). Dispositional and structural determinants of volunteerism. *Journal of Personality and Social Psychology,* 74(2), 525-537.

Perry, J.L. & Thomson, A.M. (2004). *Civic service: What difference does it make?* Armonk, NY: M.E. Sharpe, Inc.

Peter D. Hart & Associates. (1999). *The new face of retirement: Older Americans, civic engagement, and the longevity revolution* (Survey report). San Francisco: Civic ventures.

Peter D. Hart & Associates. (2002). *The new face of retirement: Older Americans, civic engagement, and the longevity revolution* (Survey report). San Francisco: Civic ventures.

Pillemer, K., Moen, P., Wethington, E., & Glasgow, N. (Eds.). (2000). *Social integration in the second half of life.* Baltimore, MD: Johns Hopkins University Press.

Polivka, L. (2001). Globalization, aging, and ethics. *Journal of Aging and Identity,* 6(3), 147-163.

Polivka, L. (2002). Globalization, aging, and ethics, part II: Toward a just global society. *Journal of Aging and Identity,* 7(3), 195-211.

Putnam, R.D. (1993). The prosperous community: Social capital and public life. *The American Prospect,* 13, 35-42.

Putnam, R.D. (2000). *Bowling alone: The collapse and revival of American community.* New York: Simon & Schuster.

Putnam, R.D. & Feldstein, L.M. (2003). *Better together: Restoring the American community.* New York: Simon & Schuster.

Rich, P. (1999). American voluntarism, social capital, and political culture. *Annals of the American Academy of Political and Social Science,* 565, 15-34.

Riley, M.W. & Riley, J.W., Jr. (1994). Age integration and the lives of older people. *The Gerontologist,* 34(1), 110-115.

Robert, S.A. (2002). Community context and aging: Future research issues. *Research on Aging,* 24(6), 579-599.

Rowe, J.W. & Kahn, R.L. (1998). Successful aging. *The Gerontologist,* 37(4), 433-440.

Sainer, J.S. (1976). The community cares: Older volunteers. *Social Policy,* 73-75.

Salamon, L.M., Anheier, H.K., List, R., Toepler, S., Sokolowski, S.W., & Associates. (1999). *Global civil society: Dimensions of the nonprofit sector.* Baltimore, MD: The Johns Hopkins Center for Civil Society Studies.

Salamon, L.M. & Sokolowski, W. (2001). *Volunteering in cross-national perspective: Evidence from 24 countries.* Working Paper No. 40. The Johns Hopkins Comparative Nonprofit Sector Project. Baltimore, MD: The Johns Hopkins Center for Civil Society Studies.

Sanchez-Jankowski, M. (2002). Minority youth and civic engagement: The impact of group relations. *Applied Developmental Science,* 6(4), 237-245.

Schaie, K.W. (1998). *Methodological issues in aging research.* New York: Springer.

Schudson, J. (1996). What if civic life didn't die? *American Prospect,* 25 (March-April), 17-20.

Schuller, T. (2000). Social and human capital: The search for appropriate techno-methodology. *Policy Studies,* 21(1), 25-35.

Second World Assembly on Ageing. (2002). Building a society for all ages. Madrid, Spain. Available online at http://www.un.org/ageing/prkit/productiveageing .htm.

Settersten, R.A., Jr. & Hagestad, G.O. (1996). What's the latest? II. Cultural age deadlines for educational and work transitions. *The Gerontologist,* 36(5), 602-613.

Sherraden, M. (2001). *Civic service: Issues, outlook, institution building, perspective*. St. Louis: Center for Social Development, Washington University.

Sherraden, M., Sherraden, M.S., & Eberly, D. (1990). Comparing and understanding non-military service in different nations. In D. Eberly and M. Sherraden (Eds.), *The moral equivalent of war? A study of non-military service in nine nations* (pp. 154-190). Westport, CT: Greenwood Press.

Social Security Administration (SSA). (1999). *Social Security programs throughout the world: 1999*. SSA Publication No. 13-11805. Washington, DC: SSA.

Stolle, D. (1998). Bowling together, bowling alone: The development of generalized trust in voluntary associations. *Political Psychology*, 19, 497-525.

Tang, F., McBride, A.M., and Sherraden, M. (2003). *Toward measurement of civic service*. Research background paper. St. Louis: Center for Social Development, Washington University.

Tapia, M.N. (2003). "Servicio" and "solidaridad" in South American Spanish. In H. Perold, S. Stroud, & M. Sherraden (Eds.), *Service enquiry: Service in the 21st century* (pp. 139-149). Johannesburg: comPress.

Thoits, P.A. & Hewitt, L.N. (2001). Volunteer work and well-being. *Journal of Health and Social Behavior*, 42, 115-131.

Torney-Purta, J. (2002). The school's role in developing civic engagement: A study of adolescents in twenty-eight countries. *Applied Developmental Science*, 6(4), 203-212.

U.S. Bureau of Labor Statistics. (2003). *Volunteering in the United States, 2003*. Available online at http://www.bls.gov/news.release/volun.nr0.htm.

Uhlenberg, P. (1992). Population aging and social policy. *Annual Review of Sociology*, 18, 449-474.

United Nations. (2002a). *International year of volunteers: Outcomes and future perspectives*. New York: United Nations.

United Nations. (2002b). *Population ageing 2002*. New York: United Nations.

United Nations Development Programme. (1999). *Human development report*. New York: Oxford University Press.

United Nations Volunteer Programme. (2001). *Expert working group meeting on volunteering and social development*. New York: United Nations.

Van Willigen, M. (2000). Differential benefits of volunteering across the life course. *Journals of Gerontology: Social Sciences*, 55B(5), S308-S318.

Wilson, J. (2000). Volunteering. *Annual Review of Sociology*, 26, 215-240.

Wilson, J. & Musick, M. (1998). The contribution of social resources to volunteering. *Social Science Quarterly*, 79(4), 799-814.

Wuthnow, R. (1999). Mobilizing civic engagement: The changing impact of religious involvement. In M. Fiorina and T. Skocpol (Eds.), *Civic engagement in American democracy* (pp. 331-363). Washington, DC: Brookings Institution.

Chapter 12

Civic Engagement Research, Policy, and Practice Priority Areas: Future Perspectives on the Baby Boomer Generation

Laura B. Wilson
Sharon P. Simson

INTRODUCTION

The future of civic engagement by the baby boomer generation is rooted in today's knowledge, innovations, and actions. As we have seen from the preceding chapters, there is still much to understand and much to be done to create a framework for what active engagement of the fifty-plus population will look like over the next thirty years. With unknowns regarding income, employment, lifestyle choices, and variations within the boomer generation itself, looking toward the next steps requires a multifaceted approach with numerous perspectives.

To envision priority areas for future research, policy, and best practices regarding civic engagement in later life, we asked civic engagement leaders in eight key government programs, nonprofit agencies, and foundations for their perspectives about this question: *What are your or your agency's priority areas for research, policy, and best practices for the next five years regarding civic engagement and the baby boomer generation?*

Future perspectives were offered by leaders of these key organizations: AARP, the Administration on Aging of the Department of Health and Human Services, the Corporation for National and Community Service, Generations United, the Gerontological Society of

America, the Harvard School of Public Health/MetLife Foundation, the National Council on Aging, the Points of Light Foundation, and the Robert Wood Johnson Foundation. The responses of each agency are summarized. Each response is presented separately in order to provide the reader with an understanding of individual and organizational perspectives.

ADMINISTRATION ON AGING

United States Department of Health and Human Services, Washington, DC
Carol Crecy, MBA, Director, Center for Communication and Consumer Services

Volunteers are an integral part of all the programs of the Administration on Aging. Although we don't collect data on the number of volunteers we have in all the older Americans Act programs, we estimate about 500,000 volunteers across the country.

I want to talk about how the Older Americans Act uses volunteers to help provide services to older Americans through four of our programs: nutrition, the long-term care ombudsman, Senior Medicare Patrol Project, and transportation. I am going to provide snapshots of a few programs of the many, many more out there.

In our nutrition program many of the people who deliver meals to homebound seniors are, in fact, seniors themselves. In the congregate meals sites a lot of the people who prepare or serve meals are volunteers and seniors themselves.

The long-term care ombudsman program has advocates for older persons and the person's family who help resolve problems in nursing homes, board and care homes, and assisted living facilities. We have specific information that in 2002 we had about 10,800 volunteers; 8,200 of them were certified to investigate complaints.

For the Senior Medicare Patrol Project we have been partners with the Center for Medicare and Medicaid Services and the Department of Human Service's Office of the Inspector General to help fight fraud, error, and abuse in the Medicare and Medicaid programs. The Medicare Patrols are retired professionals who agree to become volunteers. They help people read their Medicare summary notices, look for fraud, and work with Medicare providers on potential errors that have been discovered. In 2003, the last year for which we have numbers for them, the project trained over 7,500 seniors volunteers who educated over 467,000 Medicare beneficiaries. Over the past six years, we believe that we have trained over 40,000 volunteers to serve in this program.

Transportation is the second largest service, after the nutrition program, provided under the OAA. Many of the people who are driving vans and providing transportation at the local level are volunteers. Although recently it has been difficult for volunteers to continue due to increases in gas prices, we still have a dedicated cadre of volunteers still working at the state and local level with our transportation programs.

In addition to these four programs, we have, on occasion, funded specific volunteer activities through our discretionary grants program. Around 2003 we provided funding for a new advertising campaign that was designed to recruit thousands of older Americans to participate in tutoring and mentoring programs sponsored by Experience Corps.

From a policy standpoint, volunteers are an integral part of what we do. We would not be able to reach as many people as we do if we did not have volunteers in our programs. We will continue to look for ways to strengthen the opportunities for volunteers in programs and to provide training to them and the projects themselves about how to use, recognize, and support volunteers. I cannot say enough about how very, very vital and important they are.

We conducted a survey about why older persons volunteered and what caused them to volunteer. The finding that was most striking to me was that they wanted to be asked. There are many, many people out there who have volunteer skills and abilities that could be tapped but people haven't asked them. People are looking for someone to say, "We need you. Will you come to work with us?" They also want to do something meaningful and not just "stuff envelopes." They also want a specific time frame for what they are going to be doing and how much time it is going to take. Our resource centers provide training about how to use volunteers so that they don't burn out, how to get the best use out of people, and how to place them appropriately in the right kind of volunteer assignments. Sometimes there is a misconception that there is no work involved with volunteers. That is totally incorrect. There is a lot of work in the care and feeding of the volunteer workforce. You have to have someone who pays attention to that. The Administration on Aging provides training to volunteers and to the programs that use volunteers on how to recruit and retain them. We feel that recognition is important so we encourage state and local entities to recognize volunteers.

I think the boomers are a different breed of cat. As opposed to some of the current older individuals, boomers will be more aggressive and search for volunteer opportunities. They will look at rounding out their activities. I think boomers will be working longer. They are in better health and better educated. They are not interested in retirement where you get in the Winnebago and go down to Florida. As they think about next phases of their lives, they are going to look for how to include civic engagement as part of what they do.

Boomers will look for volunteer opportunities that match what they do in their work lives. They will take the skills and abilities they used in work and translate them to volunteer opportunities. For example, if you were an accountant in your work life, you are going to look for how to take those skills to a small organization that might need help in getting their books together. They will be looking for short-term commitments and a variety of volunteer opportunities as opposed to joining up to be a volunteer at an organization and doing that for the rest of their lives.

Individual choice will determine the types of areas and organizations in which boomers might volunteer. For example, there won't be a push to work only with children or seniors, or only through religious organizations. How you live your life and what you were associated with throughout your life will be extended into the volunteer opportunities you choose as you grow older. People will go to things with which they are most familiar. If you are very active with your church while you are working, that becomes a potential opportunity for volunteering in the future. You might take on different responsibilities because you have more time than when you were working.

I'd like to see more volunteer opportunities in the future because a large group of boomers are coming down the pike who could be volunteers. I'm just playing the numbers games and thinking that way will be opened for more volunteer activities because there will be more of them. Organizations that use volunteers as an integral part of what they are doing have to change how they reach out and recruit volunteers. They can't take it for granted that this large group of baby boomers is going to come to them. Organizations have to be slicker about how they market their volunteer opportunities to baby boomers. They have to provide a variety of choices and a variety of times. They need to offer volunteer opportunities that boomers think are meaningful and not something they would think of as "envelope stuffing." Obviously you need people to stuff envelopes but they don't want that to be their only task.

The reasons why someone volunteers is so personal. I think volunteering will be related to something that happened to them in their personal lives. For example, if you had a close friend who died of breast cancer, you might become a volunteer to encourage women to get mammograms. It's the personal connection to something in your life history.

It will be important to make volunteers understand what the larger issue is and what you and your organization are trying to do with it. A volunteer needs to know that what they are doing is helping a bigger cause. It is necessary to show that linkage to the bigger issue and how their contribution fits into the bigger picture in making a difference.

Volunteerism is a very rewarding part of life and I would highly recommend it to anyone.

AARP

Washington, DC
John Rother, JD, Director of Policy and Strategy

AARP is deeply committed to promoting expanded civic engagement as a matter of healthy aging and livable communities. We have an extensive research effort ongoing to help us achieve these goals. Our efforts will focus on the following:

- Promoting a wide range of volunteer service participation including intergenerational mentoring
- Promoting healthy aging practices at the community level (physical activity, health promotion programs)
- Promoting mechanisms to support independence and functional supports for those with disabilities (including mobility options and services)
- Support of family and community-based caregiving

Our research consists of public opinion polling, small focus group research, best practices survey, and program evaluation studies. The AARP Public Policy Institute does a wide range of policy-related research and the Knowledge Management staff handles internal polling and program evaluation studies.

CORPORATION FOR NATIONAL
AND COMMUNITY SERVICE

Washington, DC
Tess Scannell, Director, Senior Corps

Senior Corps, along with a lot of other organizations, has been looking at the difference in civic engagement by people who are becoming fifty now compared to twenty to thirty years ago. Senior Corps was started thirty to forty years ago. The structure, kinds of assignments, and incentives for civic engagement are based on what was attractive to people of the WWII generation. Today, the people who are turning fifty-five to fifty-nine, the earliest of the baby boomers, have a very different idea of what will satisfy them in terms of civic engagement.

We are in the process of rethinking the ways we are looking at civic engagement for boomers even with respect to the language we use. We know we need new names for programs and new words to describe people age 50+. Retired, seniors, and volunteers no longer work. The title, Senior Corps, is not going to work. It is difficult to get around the title, Senior Companions, although we could call them caregivers. Foster grandparents—nobody wants to think of themselves as grandparents. Others have looked at this problem as well and everyone seems to be stumped when it comes to real suggestions for new language.

One way to mitigate this problem for RSVP is to take away the words behind the letters. Instead of Retired Senior Volunteer Program, the letters RSVP are compelling. For some, the word "volunteer" means that it is not as valuable as paid work. Most boomers think about volunteering as something their mothers did in the 1950s. We find that men in particular are not attracted to the idea of being a volunteer. People like doing pro bono work. The idea of a "pro bono" contribution is more attractive than volunteering. It is also necessary to offer a much wider range of roles for people and offer them roles/capacities and engage them in helping to recruit others and doing training and fund-raising.

Means testing is another issue that we think is an outdated idea. Two of the Senior Corps programs are means tested and require participants to meet income eligibility to qualify. We'd like to see that removed to make the program universal and offer the stipend to those who commit to intensive service, that is, fifteen hours per week or more. The idea of being poor in order to serve seems like an anachronism. The stipend, $2.65/hour for twenty hours of service is intended to help defray the cost of volunteering. It doesn't reflect the value of their service and isn't going to alleviate poverty.

In the early 1990s, we launched a demonstration that combined the best elements of our three programs into a new model called Experience Corps. We took the intensive service of fifteen to twenty hours a week in a service area and the stipend of Foster Grandparents and Senior Companions and married them with the "no means" test of RSVP. We found in one state who kept records that with income guidelines removed, 75 percent of the people recruited would have qualified under old guidelines and the other 25 percent were only marginally above income guidelines. Although we were not able to do much experimenting with other incentives, we think it would be a good thing to do. It would be wonderful if we could incorporate the lessons we have learned from our demonstrations back into our three regular programs. Fortunately, the Experience Corps has continued to flourish and grow using private funding.

It is important to promote civic engagement while people are still in the workplace. Volunteering is the highest in the population aged forty-five to fifty-five. It drops until age sixty when it picks up again. The latest data from AARP show that if you want to get people to volunteer, you have to get them when they are still working. People who are totally removed from the workplace are harder to lure back into civic engagement. We also know that unlike the previous population, baby boomers are not going to work until age sixty-two and then stop. They are going to be working differently and combine part-time work with service and leisure. Civic engagement can be appealing to people not connected to the workforce because it provides social interaction. People love to get together with their friends. There is a trend emerging of taking vacations to do service projects at home or in other countries.

This generation has tended not to join traditional organizations as their parents did. They want to be engaged in issues that they care about. It's going to be important to entice them into civic engagement by tapping into that interest, whether it's the environment, education, working with children or prisoners, or some other area. We need to tap into whatever they have a passion for. They need to know they are going to make a difference through civic engagement. Research shows they are not going to volunteer just for the sake of volunteering. They will be civically engaged and unpaid and devote time if it is an issue they care about and where they will make a huge difference.

Business and industry are also supporting civic engagement. For example, *Business Strengthening America* is a group of corporations that are forming partnerships with nonprofits and encouraging their workforces to volunteer and take on particular causes such as homeland security. There are all kinds of incentives for businesses to encourage their employees to get involved: (1) it is good public relations, (2) it builds teams and camaraderie in their own workforce by getting people engaged in a project beyond their work, and (3) corporations want to be good citizens. Being a good citizen is also being a good businessperson.

We think it is important for government and the private sector to devote resources to find out what will entice baby boomers to become and stay engaged. What will be the incentives for civic engagement? We want to know if a monetary incentive is what it takes to get baby boomers to serve intensively, even though they are not low income. We have a hunch that if you want people to serve more than ten to fifteen hours/week, you need to give them some kind of incentive for engagement, including small monetary incentives or tax relief. Is it frequent flier miles, prescription drug coverage, health insurance, membership in a health club? Baby boomers are going to come from all kinds of economic backgrounds. What will it take to become civically engaged with a nonprofit instead of taking a second job like going to a "big box" store and being a greeter to supplement income?

We want to expand our policies and revamp our legislative authority to enable us to tap into the large number of people who are fifty-five-plus. We want to encourage nonprofits to use our Web-based system to recruit volunteers age fifty and over. This site not only recruits people for our three programs but also provides nonprofits who might not be sponsoring one of our programs with opportunities to recruit people.

Nonprofits have to learn to accept the boomers into larger roles and take advantage of their talents. On one hand, agencies may be losing a lot of envelope stuffers but they may gain people who could help them with something such as strategic planning. To think that an agency always has to hire a consultant when it could retain a retired or semiretired or a working person over fifty who would love to use their skills to benefit their favorite environmental or youth group. All of us would be willing to stuff an envelope now and then if we knew we were taken seriously.

The future role of volunteers and volunteering needs to be redefined and resold to the upcoming population of boomers and the nonprofit organizations who can benefit from their experience, their passion, and their energy.

GENERATIONS UNITED

Washington, DC
Donna Butts, Executive Director

At Generations United we are focusing and will continue to focus on promoting intergenerational programs and connections. We want to make sure that our younger and oldest generations have voices and are active in the affairs of their communities and country. We are working in a number of ways.

We have started work on intergenerational environment programs. We have just published a new workbook and we are hoping to focus on training and the dissemination of the guide. There has been and continues to be great interest in intergenerational programs that protect the environment and make sure that the environment is in a good place to pass on to the next generation. The boomers are very involved with that. Depending on funding, we are hoping to provide seed grants to start programs as well as to promote programs through conferences and speaking engagements.

There are also a number of communities in which we are promoting intergenerational dialogues. The community brings together different generations around a specific topic or issue. Examples might be the environment or how to increase the number of voters in that town, how to address an issue such as parks and community facilities. They come together for intergenerational dialogue and visioning sessions and then continue to be involved.

An example of intergenerational cooperation is in Falcon Heights, Minnesota, just outside the Twin Cities. The mayor wanted to have an intergenerational community so the city changed the applications forms used when people want to use city property. Anybody who wants to use a city facility has to answer a questionnaire about how many generations are going to be involved. The mayor made a commitment that both older and younger people should be intentionally appointed to boards and commissions.

We monitor policy to identify opportunities for intergenerational approaches. For example, the original legislation for after-school programs didn't include older adults as one of the options for people volunteering or employed in after-school programs. We worked to make sure that older adults and intergenerational programs were included in the legislation that was passed. We think that older adults are a wonderful addition to the workforce in terms of part-time or full-time work.

We are going to continue to look for opportunities to make sure that older people are included in policies and programs. We call it barnacling. We attach the idea wherever we can. We look for both the small and large changes that need to occur. We are establishing a virtual resource center with support from Verizon where we will do a lot of online chats, provide technical assistance, and operate a program database that anyone can access.

One of the big things for the boomers is to understand that they have an obligation to younger generations to make sure they become engaged in their communities. That is something that will appeal to baby boomers who have been active all their lives. Boomers need to pass on their values, provide models, and work with future generations to be engaged in their communities.

THE GERONTOLOGICAL SOCIETY OF AMERICA

Washington, DC
Greg O'Neill, PhD, Director,
Civic Engagement in an Older America Project

In July 2004, The Gerontological Society of America (GSA) launched a five-year initiative to promote the study of civic engagement by experts in the field of aging.

With the baby boom generation on the verge of retirement, there is an increasing awareness that older adults are a growing—yet largely untapped—civic resource for responding to community needs through both paid and unpaid work. However, the aging of the baby boom generation raises questions that scholars and policymakers must address. Will civic participation increase as baby boomers move into retirement and other life demands decrease? How will women's labor force participation affect civic engagement? And what kind of programs and policies will improve the ability of older adults to participate in civic life?

Although a base of research exists that can help provide answers to such questions, scholars and policymakers are only beginning to consider how the pieces fit together. The goal of GSA's project is to stimulate research within the gerontological community that will synthesize the current state of knowledge about the impact of an aging society on civic engagement. Working together with an expert group of multidisciplinary scholars, GSA's project on "Civic Engagement in an Older America" aims to produce and promote research contributing to the development of more effective social institutions and policies that will improve the ability of older adults to participate in civic life.

The initiative, funded by a grant from The Atlantic Philanthropies, will include a series of special publications, GSA Annual Meeting symposiums, and paper awards that will culminate in a congressional briefing based on the findings of the project. In addition, the project will conduct a series of forums and focus groups across the country on the topic of civic engagement that will provide input to the 2005 White House Conference on Aging.

HARVARD SCHOOL OF PUBLIC HEALTH— METLIFE FOUNDATION INITIATIVE

Boston, MA
Susan Moses, SM, Deputy Director, Center for Health Communication and Co-Director, Harvard School of Public Health—MetLife Foundation Initiative on Retirement and Civic Engagement

The Harvard School of Public Health—MetLife Foundation Initiative on Retirement and Civic Engagement is a national media campaign to promote healthy and productive aging, reshape cultural attitudes toward the older years, and encourage boomers to share their time, skills, and experience as community volunteers. We're spotlighting the mentoring of young people as a leading example of community involvement.

The campaign is on outgrowth of our recent report, *Reinventing Aging: Baby Boomers and Civic Engagement,* published as part of Phase I of the Initiative. The report highlights key issues that must be addressed to involve large numbers of boomers in strengthening community life.

The media campaign in Phase II of the Initiative will involve a combination of news coverage, advertising, and prime-time entertainment programming to stimulate a national dialogue about the meaning and purpose of life after sixty. The average sixty-year-old today can expect to live to the age of eighty-three. This longevity revolution has created a new stage of life, nesteled between middle age and old age, from sixty to eighty. Our campaign will encourage boomers to plan for this extra decade or two of life. It will challenge them to address the question, "What will I do with the rest of my life?" by developing a "balanced portfolio" of activities that includes community involvement along with work, leisure, travel, and lifelong learning. We are all used to hearing about the need for financial planning for retirement, but we need to have a plan for how we will spend our days as well.

To address this issue, we are developming a *Guidebook for Boomers* that will present a checklist of questions that boomers can aks themselves as they develop a plan to make the most of this new stage of life. We want to encourage them to think about civic engagement—about giving back to the community as one component of a healthy lifestyle. Research has shown that there are true health benefits, both physiological and psychological, associated with staying socially engaged.

To reinvent aging, we need to tell more stories about what is possible, about how people can get involved in their community as they enter this new phase of life. We will work with journalists to stimulate ongoing coverage of productive aging, community involvement, and innovative programs that tap the talents of older boomers.

We are also working with the Hollywood creative community to encourage them to rethink and reinvent the images of aging through their storytelling. Many people believe that we, as a society, don't value older people or the experiences they have to offer. Hollywood can depict older people as being productive and contributing to society. By modeling behaviors, television and films can give viewers ideas about how positive and exciting this new stage of life can be.

We also need to create new language because the current terminology is inadequate and may, in fact, be a barrier to change. Everyone says boomers aren't going to have anything to do with the term "senior citizen," and the term "retirement" as now we know it is obsolete as well. We hope our collaboration with the Hollywood creative community can help introduce new terms into the American lexicon in the same way we did with our "Designated Driver Campaign." Writers and producers of television programs helped us introduce the concept that the driver does not drink any alcohol by incorporating the term into the scripts of shows. Three years into the campaign, the term "designated driver" was listed in the dictionary.

The leading-edge boomers came of age during the Kennedy years, when optimism and service to one's country were high on the nation's agenda. But for many boomers, the responsibilities of raising a family and andvancing their career put those ideals on hold. Now, with an extra decade or two of life, these boomers can have a second chance to fulfill those dreams. The question is, can we tap into those dormant feelings and reignite the spark? To do so, we need to create an environment that is conducive to giving back to society.

NATIONAL COUNCIL ON AGING

Washington, DC
Tom Endres, Director, Civic Engagement Initiative

The strategic plan of the National Council on Aging (NCOA) has identified three priorities it will be focusing on in the next three to five years:

1. improving the health and independence of older persons;
2. increasing the continuing contributions of older persons to their community, society, and future generations; and
3. developing caring communities.

The focus of our conversation is the second priority. NCOA has begun to move quite assertively into that area. In terms of research, our strategy is to develop new knowledge, create new ideas, and translate research into effective programs and services. We have three strategic foci.

Our first strategic focus is on innovations. We are going to be looking for emerging best practices and helping organizations develop the evidence base and the common elements of those emerging best practices. We will identify creative ideas, new knowledge, and new techniques. Once we have established the evidence base, the convincing argument that it works, and identify why it works, we will then support others in adapting that best practice.

The second strategic focus is activation. We're going to develop ways of helping others learn about the evidence supporting an emerging practice and the core elements. We will help other communities assess their readiness and resource ability to take that innovation and adapt, adopt, and replicate that best practice in their communities.

Our third area of strategic focus is advocacy. Once we know something works and why, once we have helped others successfully replicate that model or best practice, then we want to advocate for that emerging best practice so an innovation becomes adapted more widely through public policy and social change.

With regard to civic engagement, specifically, NCOA is doing a number of activities. In our RespectAbility initiative, we are conducting vigorous research with nonprofit organizations to determine their challenges, barriers, and practices in tapping older adults as a resource for their organizations. Organizations need to respect the abilities of older adults and show that respect by developing well-organized, well-led, and well-planned opportunities for attracting older adults to organizations. Older adults need to respect themselves for what they can contribute. RespectAbility is funded by the Atlantic Philanthropies and uses a three-phase process.

• First, we conducted in-depth interviews with twenty CEOs of large, national, nonprofit organizations.
• Second, we conducted focus groups in four cities across the country with eighty local affiliates of large organizations to identify the consistency between what we learn from the in-depth interviews with the national leaders and the experience of their local affiliate leaders. We acquire a national perspective and a local perspective.
• Third, we are conducting a Web-based survey of over 800 affiliate leaders across the country. This survey will provide a quantitative reference for substantiating the qualitative findings from the in-depth interviews and the focus groups.

We will take the learning from this research and develop a series of public policy briefs with recommendations for changes in two categories:

1. Changes in existing programs and policies to determine if we can make them a little more responsive to the needs of the organizations at this point in time. Can we improve what we have?
2. Institutional changes to prepare for the large number of older adults, the boomers mainly, who will be coming of age and available. We consider the structural and infrastructural needs to accommodate and attract older adults to contribute to their communities.

NCOA is establishing a process of accessing innovations and identifying the best practices of those innovations. We are developing a methodology and Web-based tool that will help others to become aware of a practice that we have found to be proven successful and the key elements necessary for success. We want to take successful innovations and help spread them to hundreds of other communities across the country.

We are interested in developing innovations ourselves. NCOA has developed an initiative, Wisdom Works, which is an innovation supported by the MetLife Foundation. Wisdom Works focuses on the development of self-managed teams. We are looking to find what older adults, when brought together, identify as their interests and needs in their local areas. We want to bring a group of people together and let them develop themselves as a self-managed team to solve community problems. Wisdom Works is important because we can develop flexible models independent of organizations. We can provide creative mechanisms that encourage older adults to get together to form a group to identify their interests and define their capabilities in order to help their community in whatever way they want.

NCOA is producing a national social marketing strategy to help publicize widely the research findings and policy changes that we will recommend from the RespectAbility initiative. This communication strategy consists of an hour-long documentary film to engage seasoned, veteran journalists to become more knowledgeable and write about this issue. An outreach effort will take segments of the documentary and conduct town hall meetings in major media markets around the country. We will engage leaders in a discussion about the aging of their communities and their challenges and opportunities. We hope to get the word out about our research that has identified problems and promising practices. We will put together resource and technical assistance materials to help organizations move in the directions they need to move if, in fact, older adults are going to be a resource to help them meet their organizational purposes.

Another practice is establishing a number of national resource centers to help coordinate, support, and spark innovation throughout the network of the hundreds of senior centers across the country. NCOA has also established a National Resource Center for Family Friends, a program that matches older adults with families that have a child with a special or exceptional need. The older adult supports the family and reduces the stress. We want to capture the best practices within these programs and develop similar programs across the country. We also administer a very large older workers program to look at how we can help develop unpaid and paid service opportunities for older folks.

We have established partnerships to work on all these programs. We work with the National Assembly of Human Services Organizations, a seventy-year-old organization. The members are the seventy largest nonprofit organizations in the country. The National Assembly has just formed a new affinity group called the Aging Caucus, a subset of national organizations interested in examining how the aging of America is affecting their organizations and, specifically, the services they provide.

It is a very exciting time. We are at a point where attention will be paid not only to concerns about health, health care costs, and services, but also to the resource potential of aging Americans.

POINTS OF LIGHT FOUNDATION

Washington, DC
Christopher Cihlar, PhD, Director of Research and Evaluation

We are not focusing significant resources on this effort although we are in the process of putting together a research proposal for this group which will be sent out in August (2004) that focuses on the health benefits of volunteering and how it impacts those approaching retirement. Basically, trying to understand first how volunteering can ease this transition and second, what, if any, health benefits (mental as well as physical) can be associated with it. This thought is the extent of our research agenda with this population at the current time.

ROBERT WOOD JOHNSON FOUNDATION

Princeton, New Jersey
Robin Mockenhaupt, PhD, MPH,
Interim Director, Health Group

The Foundation has several programs for older people to use their talents in civic engagement, the most well-known of which is Experience Corps. Experience Corps was launched as a program to mobilize older Americans to serve communities with unmet needs such as helping elementary schoolchildren improve their reading skills and helping at-risk children. The program began with five initial sites and, with funding from the Robert Wood Johnson Foundation and Atlantic Philanthropies, now counts more than 1,500 volunteers in thirteen cities throughout the country.

One main effort on civic engagement to date is the provision of several million dollars over a couple years to help Experience Corps go deeper and broader—to go deeper into cities where they have an Experience Corps component as well as to take it to other cities.

The Robert Wood Johnson Foundation focuses on health and health care. Civic engagement has been tied into the work in one of our Foundation priorities in what we call our vulnerable populations portfolio. Older adults are considered as one of the populations potentially at risk for poor health outcomes along with low-income children and families, and people with mental and physical disabilities.

There has been very little work done in the United States on public policy and civic engagement. This is an area that absolutely needs more attention. Having said that, what probably needs to come first is more research so that it can inform the public policy. On the other hand, this does not necessarily need to be sequential. Research and public policy can be happening at the same time. Good public policy should be based on well-informed and documented outcomes. We need to pay more attention to outcome research that shows us whether the investment in civic engagement programming and interventions pays off.

Solid, science-based work would make it easier to go to legislators who sometimes (and sometimes don't) use science-based work to help inform their decisions about public policies. I think that it would be great if we could get a legislator to sign onto evidence-based efforts to increase civic engagement in public policy. The way laws get made and policy gets written is when something happens to some legislator's mother or father, sister or brother or uncle. It's like making sausage. You don't really want to see how it's made. But the reality is that is how it happens. That is how it happens in disease areas. That's why NIH [National Institutes of Health] and research on every new technology are well-funded. Wouldn't it be wonderful if the mother or father of a legislator was involved in some kind of civic engagement program and the legislator used it as an example of why we should have more civic engagement programs? Maybe that's an angle, too, that we should be paying more attention to. So, hey, let's do that with civic engagement.

This may sound simple but we need more civic engagement programming and interventions. There are wonderful examples but there aren't enough of them. We need to continue to make progress on this area. I think the current boomers and the next generation after that will push for this to happen. It's great that there is consumer demand for civic engagement and that is what is going to drive it. We should just keep on plugging away at ways to accelerate and respond to that demand. To accomplish this, we need to get some more solid research done and we need to talk to policymakers.

CONCLUSION

The perspectives of these government, nonprofit, and foundation leaders regarding civic engagement and the baby boomer generation validate the policy, research, and best practice findings of the previous chapters in this book. Perhaps the most significant theme is the need to prepare for the baby boomers both in terms of what the baby boomers will expect from volunteer service opportunities and how non-profit organizations might need to adapt in order to work effectively with this generation of potential volunteers.

What does this mean from policy, practice, and research perspectives? Our experts concur that meaningful volunteer roles need to be designed and implemented and that more and better roles are going to be essential. The experts also validate the need for new language for the term "volunteering" and testing new incentives that might encourage participation. Experts agree that it is essential for the media to be involved and committed to presenting public information about civic engagement. This media involvement entails a two-part approach. First, the fifty-plus population needs to be made aware of new and developing opportunities in which they might invest their energy and time. Second, the public and nonprofits, in particular, need to be made aware of the extensive skills and capacities of the coming generation of baby boomers. As a result, they will need to adjust their thinking about what is possible in both paid and unpaid work to take advantage of this resource.

A clear message in the interview responses is that if nonprofits continue to do what worked in the past to attract volunteers, their methods are not likely to be effective with the boomers. The degree to which changes are possible or those that will yield the best results are only now emerging. The respondents point to research, infrastructure changes, and partnerships with business and communities as avenues that are being or need to be explored.

The conclusion of all the preceding work is that the state of knowledge about civic engagement and the baby boomers is still in an early stage of development. There is still much to be done in terms of research, policy, and practice to ensure maximizing the potential impact that baby boomers can have on community needs. Current innovative opportunities need to be broadly and deeply infused throughout the United States. Numerous new approaches to involving the boomers must emerge from conversations with all sectors including the boomers themselves, businesses, and nonprofit organizations.

No amount of innovation and media attention will be worthwhile if nonprofit organizations are not adequately prepared to meet these new challenges. Changing the way in which organizations work with volunteers will change not only the nature of volunteerism but also entire organizational infrastructures. Researchers, policymakers, and practitioners must consider integrated holistic approaches to respond to this emerging area of civic engagement in order to achieve a balanced outcome that is beneficial to the volunteer, the nonprofit organization and its clients, and to the community.

These new approaches must be adequately evaluated for effectiveness to demonstrate their impact. The future capacity of our society to meet human needs in the coming decades may depend on our success in strengthening, upgrading, integrating, and evaluating new ideas and innovations that advance civic engagement by the baby boomer generation.

Index

Page numbers followed by the letter "f" indicate figures; and those followed by the letter "t" indicate tables.